Courageous Conversations on Dying

The Gift of Palliative Care

**A Practical Guide for Physicians,
Healthcare Providers,
and All the People They Serve**

Shahid Aziz, MD

Copyright © 2018 by Shahid Aziz. All rights reserved. With the exception of short quotations for articles and reviews, no part of this publication may be reproduced, transmitted, scanned, distributed, stored in any form or by any means, electronic, mechanical, photocopying, recording, or otherwise, without prior written permission from the author.

DISCLAIMER:
Nothing in this book should be taken as legal advice. Please check your local laws.

Patient stories are true but names and minor details are changed for confidentiality.

Shahid Aziz, MD

Email: askdraziz@gmail.com
Twitter: @hospicedocaziz
Blog: you deserve a good death.blogspot.com

Published in the United States of America.

ISBN 978-1983403286

Cover art: Shahid Aziz, MD
Cover design: Maureen Ryan Griffin, wordplaynow.com

ADVANCE PRAISE for *COURAGEOUS CONVERSATIONS ON DYING*

"**Dr. Aziz unpacks what good end-of-life care looks like and what clinicians (doctors in particular) should do to best support each patient and those grieving that patient's death.** His poignant stories, case examples, and practical tips help de-mystify "advance care planning," described as 'probably one of the best gifts one can give to one's children and loved ones.' This book is a gift as well — to those who provide patient care and those who educate and train health care providers. Since good end-of-life care benefits not just the patient but all who live with memories of the patient's final days, it's a gift that can keep on giving."

- Anita Tarzian, PhD, RN, Program Coordinator, Maryland Health Care Ethics Committee Network (MHECN), Associate Professor, U of Maryland School of Nursing

"**Although we communicate with patients all the time, rarely do we as physicians know how to actually 'do' it.** We tend to talk a lot, filling the silence, and not listen effectively. These are skills generally not taught in medical training. Dr. Aziz gives medical practitioners practical advice and scripts to use on a daily basis for those we truly 'care' for, our patients."

- Geoffrey Coleman MD, MHA, Chief Medical Officer, Montgomery Hospice/Palliative Medicine Consultants

"In *Courageous Conversations on Dying*, Dr. Aziz has distilled his years of work with seriously ill patients and their families in complex decision-making. The insights gained from that experience and his review of the work and practice of a wide range of contemporary palliative practitioners makes this book a worthwhile read."

- Christopher D Kearney MD, Medical Director MedStar Health Palliative Care

"What a lovely gift Dr. Aziz has given the world with his *Courageous Conversations*. Grounded in best practices and a lifetime of experience, Dr. Aziz's book is chock-a-block with examples and sample conversations to gentle the end of life experience. He gently leads the reader by the hand on this learning journey. The quotes sprinkled throughout are keepers, worthy of daily reflection. Thank you, Dr. Aziz!"

- Mary Lynn McPherson, PharmD, MA, MDE, BCPS, CPE, Executive Director Advanced Post-Graduate Education in Palliative Care

DEDICATION

This book is a humble effort to impart what I have learned from my parents, my patients and their families, my colleagues, family, friends, and teachers. I dedicate it to them all.

May it help others to achieve a peaceful end to this wonderful life for themselves, their loved ones, and for those in their care.

CONTENTS

Preface 11

Introduction 15

1 | Talking About the End – Why Is It So Hard? 19

2 | Accepting Death – A Personal Story 25

3 | The Gift 29

4 | Describing Palliative Care and Hospice Care 33

5 | Communication – The Key to Good Palliative Care, Resolving Conflicts and Misunderstandings 39

6 | Basic Rules for Having Courageous Conversations and Giving "Bad News" 45

7 | The Power of Touch 55

8 | The Power of Prayer 57

9 | Realistic Hope 59

10 | The Ethical Question for The Physician 61

11 | Advance Care Planning for End of Life (EOL) in the *Inpatient* Setting – "The Three Questions" to Establish Minimum Goals of Living: A Way to Set Minimum Thresholds for Supporting Life by Artificial Means 63

12 | Advance Care Planning for End of Life (EOL) and "The Three Questions" in the *Outpatient* Setting 85

13 | Creating A Document of ACP/Advance Directive 99

14 | Examples of End of Life Living Goals and Plans 103

15 | Preparing for Dementia – The Slow Downward Spiral 107

16 | Making Difficult Choices: Whose Responsibility Is It? – Decision vs Recommendation vs Recommended Decision 111

17 | Helping Surrogates Make Decisions 123

18 | Listening and Empathy: The Glue That Binds Us! 131

19 | Building Trust 135

20 | Managing Cross-Cultural Issues 137

21 | Addressing DNR/DNAR 145

22 | Making the Futility Talk with Patient and Family Easier – The Futility Graph as a Visual Tool 153

23 | Additional Visual Tools That Enhance Communication 159

24 | Envelope DNAR/Pocket DNAR For Children 161

25 | The Hard Talks with Parents and Children 163

26 | Cutting to the Chase – Clinical Ethical Decision-Making: The Fastest Way to Come to the Best Decision for the Highest Good 169

27 | Goals and The Quality of Life 171

28 | Further Examples of End of Life Living Goals and Plans 173

29 | Words, Words, Words 183

30 | Lessons Learned – A Round-Up of Tips and Insights from Physicians and Palliative Care Team Members 193

31 | Physician-Assisted Suicide/Physician-Assisted Dying/Aid in Dying/Death with Dignity 205

32 | Beware of Burnout 211

33 | Reflections on Death and Dying 213

Appendix: Form: My End of Life Goals and Plans 219

In Gratitude 221

About the Author 223

PREFACE

Having suffered along with the suffering of others, both patients, their families, and my family, I am convinced that courageous conversations on death and dying, including end of life wishes and minimum acceptable goals of living, need to occur now, while one still has decision-making capacity.

It's time to stop supporting the public's unrealistic expectations of what medicine can do. Realistic, candid discussions will help patients and families gain the understanding necessary to accept death with less fear and anxiety. **Death needs to be talked about as part of life**, just as any other fearful topic, such as sex, drugs, debt, money, or addiction.

Why is it necessary to talk about end of life issues while one may be in good health?

One of the major reasons is that **we have no guarantee that tomorrow we will still be able to make our own decisions.** One's capacity to make decisions can be lost in a flash from trauma or disease. There is no question that the end is coming and all of us will have to eventually embark on this journey. So an important question for all of us is, how do we best prepare for this voyage?

Most Americans want to die at home, but at least one third of all deaths occur in short-stay hospitals. According to the Dartmouth Institute for Health Policy and Clinical Practice, out of the nearly $700 billion annual Medicare budget about one-third is spent in the last six months of one's life.

According to the National Center for Health Statistics those dying in hospital stay about three days longer (average 7.9 days) compared to all other admissions (4.8 days). Many of these people are hooked to machines or undergoing aggressive therapies – not a very gentle or dignified end. Thus, **the sooner we have these conversations the better, and definitely better late than never.**

My professional journey took me from academic pediatrics to medical ethics chair, where I was presented with one ethical dilemma after another that had to do with end of life issues. Most of the consults came from the adult ICU. I saw how poorly we handled end of life and how much suffering there was on all sides, including the healthcare workers.

This propelled me towards working on end of life issues, gaining experience and expertise in hospice and palliative medicine, starting the palliative care program at our local hospital, helping start the pediatric hospice services at the local hospice, and finally doing my boards in Hospice and Palliative Medicine.

All my work now is with children and adults with life-limiting illnesses. Most of my time is spent in advance care planning, helping patients and families make difficult decisions based on rational choices. I also spend a fair amount of time teaching lay people the need for advance care planning, advance directives, and related end of life issues.

Because of my love of teaching, I also continue to teach medical ethics and palliative medicine, along with care planning for end of life to medical students and healthcare providers.

This book is a concerted effort to impart what I have learned in a practical format. I do owe thanks to all who have helped me learn, including the students for asking the tough questions – and to you, the reader, who will carry this knowledge to those in need of it.

Working together, we can decrease suffering and make the end of life a little smoother, a little more dignified, a little more rational, a little more caring, a little more loving, and a little more peaceful for all concerned.

I am convinced that decisions at the end of life would be much easier and the cost would be much lower if every person had their goals and a plan for living near end of life laid out ahead of time.

It is up to us, all the physicians and healthcare workers, especially those in the palliative care world, to come up with ways to make this happen.

References:

1. http://www.dartmouthatlas.org/keyissues/issue.aspx?con=29
2. NCHC Data Brief No. 118, March 2013

Advance Care Planning
is the key
to decreasing suffering
at the end of life
for all concerned

INTRODUCTION

This book is a practical guide for physicians and healthcare workers on how to have conversations on death and dying and related end of life issues. It can also be very helpful to patients and general public.

This includes not only holding caring conversations when one is faced with **giving "bad news," but also** having those initial and ongoing conversations that guide and support patients and families in preparing for the end of life and its management. This can ensure a meaningful life and a good death for the patient and peace for the families. This involves **advance care planning,** not just for the ill but also as part of anticipatory guidance for the well.

We all deserve a wonderful life, one enriched with family, friends, and the ability to live according to our own hopes, wishes, and desires. This can also include a good, dignified, and peaceful death.

Death is a part of everyone's life and *a good death* can be a very real part of anyone's life. But it takes timely and focused planning in advance. Physicians can help their patients tremendously in this regard by approaching this subject with care and courage early on.

We make choices every day on how we wish to live and what principles are important to us. We can also extend that thinking to include the choice to prepare for death in a proactive fashion so that we die with as much peace and dignity as possible. Let us call it our "End of Life Living

Plan." Or even better, our "End of Life Living AND Dying Plan."

There are two important realizations necessary in order to put together a successful living and dying plan:
1) You must complete it before you actually need it.
2) There is a 100% chance that you will need it.

Once you embrace these key truths, you can begin to make plans. It is probably safe to say that the majority of us put these plans off until it is too late. We must break this trend.

Would you take a vacation without making plans? A trip to another country? Probably not. Most of the time we do not make a trip to the grocery store without making a plan. Then why are we not planning for this inevitable trip?

The end is not known, cannot be predicted, and will most likely arrive when we do not expect it. But arrive it will. We need to prepare well for it and help our patients and families do the same.

Technology has propelled us into the marvel of never imagined wonderful and amazing life-saving and life-prolonging treatments. What state of existence these may sometimes leave us in is another story. Unfortunately, many a time it is an existence that sustains a poor quality of life.

Take the case of Margie, who at the age of 67, with longstanding diabetes and two earlier strokes, was admitted in respiratory failure from severe pneumonia and sepsis. She was aggressively treated with antibiotics and artificial ventilation. Unable to be weaned off the respirator, she was moved to a long-term vent unit on trach, and a PEG in an unconscious state. She remained that way for over two months, also receiving dialysis for renal failure, and developed over 20 skin ulcers. After multiple meetings with the family, and just short of getting a court order to stop life-sustaining treatments, the family finally agreed to take her off the vent and dialysis and let her die in peace. Not quite the peaceful dignified death we would hope for.

As physicians, we could have made her end of life appreciably better if we had approached the end of life issues much earlier on in the process, preferably while she still had her capacity to make her own decisions.

This book concerns itself mainly with just that important aspect: **our role of guiding patients through their decision-making for end of life, concentrating on the minimum acceptable goals for living.**

When talking with patients and families about end of life issues, we must acquire the skills to guide them. These skills can be learned, as explained in the coming pages. You'll gain the knowledge of how to prepare for these conversations, including what kind of setting, what words to use, how to be a good listener, how to empathize, how to help in decision-making, how to support the patient and family in planning ahead for end of life issues, and more, along with many case studies to illustrate the points.

To find what constitutes meaningful existence at a minimal level for a given person may involve a multitude of dialogues handled with skill – the chapters that follow will give you all you need to hold these conversations.

It takes courage and compassion to talk about death and dying with an ill patient who has come to you looking for help – wanting to get better, get cured, and live long.

At the same time, even more courage is necessary when planning ahead and discussing the end of life with patients who are well. We will explore strategies for both situations in **"Advance Care Planning"** and **"The Three Questions."**

As physicians and healthcare providers, it is our responsibility to initiate these conversations with our patients. **If we keep waiting for the patient to initiate these conversations ("when he is ready, he will ask"), I fear we will miss the opportunity while he/she has the capacity to make decisions.**

If the patient loses the ability to make his or her own decisions, we will be in the more difficult scenario of having to guide and decide with their surrogates. Strategies on how to work with them will also be explored in **"Helping Surrogates Make Decisions."**

1 | TALKING ABOUT THE END – WHY IS IT SO HARD?

Death is the "D" word society has avoided. Perhaps it will not happen if we don't talk about it? Maybe there is something you know that you are not disclosing, since you are talking about the possibility of death?

Families are afraid to anger or upset each other and so avoid the subject of death. To patients who are well, this is even more of a heavy discussion than when there is a serious, life-limiting illness.

Life is precious. Under most circumstances, no one wants it to end. As modern medicine keeps helping us to live longer, deep down we start thinking perhaps, maybe just this once, a miracle will happen. But when it doesn't, we become resolved, at the very least, to slow the inevitable as we cling to this life, many times with more suffering.

The fascinating innovations in medicine and technology are helping us to live longer with great results. Just look at how respirators, transplants, dialysis, defibrillators, and artificial kidneys and hearts have extended the lives of our patients. However, with these impressive medical technologies, **we are also extending how long some of our patients suffer their marginal existence as chronic disease slowly marches them toward the bitter end**. At times when patients with the capacity to do so have made clear, reasoned choices, it may be rational to provide such aggressive therapies. **Thus, there is the need for timely talks and discussions with each individual** about their values, wishes and, goals of living near the end of life. **Time and timeliness is of the essence here.**

In healthcare, we are using a lot of our resources in the last six to twelve months of a patient's life. These resources can be substantially reduced by eliminating unnecessary treatments and tests. This can be achieved if everyone has a written advance care plan that makes their goals and wishes known.

Whenever I consult on a patient who has capacity for decision-making, he/she invariably makes more reasonable and rational choices than when family members are making decisions.

First, we have to accept death as a natural part of life. Then perhaps we can also talk about it realistically. Death is a difficult topic to discuss, since it is often considered negative. Talking about potentially hurtful end of life issues oftentimes makes death real and exacerbates the fear that it may soon come.

But death does always eventually come. And just thinking and talking about it can make patients and their loved ones very unhappy, troubled, and morose about the coming inevitable loss and grief. Sad as it may be, death is a part of life, a continuum without which life is not complete.

Physicians also have a very hard time talking about the possibility of death. Patients are looking to get better and live longer, not to be told the opposite and be "given up upon."

There are many reasons why physicians may be reluctant in taking part in serious end of life discussions and decisions.

These include not knowing what to say, unpredictability of prognosis, avoidance of conflict, fear of law suits, unfamiliarity of the law and skepticism of institutional support.

As physicians and caregivers, *we* have to accept death, not as a bad ending, but as a part of life. Our ability to discuss it with our patients demonstrates a growth of our understanding and our recognition of the necessity to discuss it at the appropriate time. We can celebrate our having achieved the knowledge to help the patient and the family through this very emotional but unavoidable circumstance. These include not knowing what to say, unpredictability of prognosis, avoidance of conflict, fear of law suits, unfamiliarity of the law and skepticism of institutional support.

Just because we let patients die does not mean we should stop taking care of them or their loved ones, who may be dealing with the complex, and often conflicting emotions that come with the loss of a loved one. For example, in such circumstances, it's natural for family members to feel a sense of relief at the end of their loved one's suffering. This relief can be confusing. We can offer our reassurance that this is very normal and common.

As a matter of fact, the patient and his or her family will now need more attention and time from their medical team, throughout the dying process and beyond.

The good news is that, as healthcare workers, we are able to cope with death and dying better when we accompany our patients through the grieving process.

I remember my residency days when, while on rounds, we would discuss terminally ill patients outside their rooms with the door closed and, many times, not even go in to talk to them. Now, as a hospice and palliative care physician, I get to openly talk about the end of life with patients, families, children, and parents alike (since I do pediatric palliative and hospice care as well as adult). **I go to funerals. It is one of the best things I do that affirm my role as the physician I studied to be, to help others in their moment of need.**

My patients and their families in turn make me feel fulfilled in my mission as a healer by their show of appreciation. Sure, it is hard and there are a lot of tears, but it is worth it.

Rickie died at two and a half years of age from a neurodegenerative disease. Our hospice team had been involved with his care over the last year before his death. We all got to know the family well as we spent hours at a time with them in their difficult journey. After Rickie died, the hospice team members, including myself, went to the funeral.

Their primary physicians were there too. The parents greeted all of us very warmly and were visibly happy and grateful for our presence. They acknowledged all by name and later sent our team a note which read:

Tremendous thanks for all the support you provided our family and Rickie during his final months. Through your loving care Rickie was in comfortable surroundings as he negotiated his way through the final stages of his journey. And we very much appreciate your participation in Rickie's memorial service. We thank all of you for your selfless devotion to our precious boy.

There's no lack of sad cases where patients suffered far too long with far too many non-beneficial treatments. Here are just a few representative cases I've seen:

- *A 64-year-old gentleman with end stage dementia, septic shock and DIC going to surgery for perforated bowel after two weeks in the ICU with deteriorating clinical status.*
- *A 70-year-old gentleman with multiple organ failure who was resuscitated three times over a two-week period before finally dying.*
- *A terminal patient who underwent G-tube placement three days before his death.*
- *A patient with metastatic cancer who received aggressive therapies, including his chemo, one day before death.*

These experiences go on and on. Of course, there is an occasional seriously ill patient who survives the ICU and hospital after aggressive therapies, which impacts the expectations of the general public. Most of the time, however, we can prognosticate fairly accurately which patients will not do well, especially when we have given a trial of therapies and seen poor progress.

2 | ACCEPTING DEATH – A PERSONAL STORY

I was 20 years away from becoming a palliative care physician when I began to have end of life discussions with my father. Looking back now, I am not sure that I was even aware of what I was doing at the time. But I do know that it was this experience with my father that actually taught me how to think about "goals of living at the end of life."

He called me, his son the doctor, from Pakistan to say that he was having pain in his left arm when he would go on his two-to-three-mile daily walk. He loved walking after dinner, long and fast. When I was a teenager, I would often walk with him, and it was hard for me to keep up with him.

The pain ended up being an early sign of angina, which sublingual medication helped him to cope with fairly well. He was still able to walk for miles, drive his car, and live alone.

A few years later, he called again. Now his angina was getting worse. He said his pain was now occurring when he walked about a mile, or even less, and seemed to be getting stronger.

Fearing an inevitable heart attack, I advised him that his heart vessels were probably narrowing, but that this was fixable. I urged him to come to the United States so that this could be taken care of. Otherwise, he was risking a heart attack any day.

He understood, but made excuses: It was difficult to travel. He was grateful and very happy to have lived such a wonderful life, to have seen all his children grow up, get married and have grandchildren. He was thankful to God and missed his wife, my mother who had died over ten years earlier.

"No," he said, "I am ready to go. I miss your mother. I wish to live as long as possible, but on my own, and I do not want to be dependent on anyone else. I pray to God for that every day. When my time comes, I hope he takes me quickly without dependence on others. That is my wish."

A few weeks later my wife and I were lying in bed reading when I suddenly smelled a strong sweet rose aroma. "Are you wearing perfume?" I asked my wife.

She said no.

A few moments later I again smelled the sweet odor. I again asked her if she was sure that she was not wearing perfume.

She denied it again, a little annoyed at my repetitious questioning.

That night, I dreamed I was at a hillside resort. And this wonderful man, my father, Abbajan as we used to call him, whom I loved so much, met me in a place of worship, looking marvelously healthy and at peace.

He gave me the longest embrace that I can ever remember. The next morning, I told my wife that I think my dad or perhaps both my parents had come to visit me and that I had better call home.

"Something is up with Abbajan," I said, but in my hurry to get to work I did not get to call.

Later that day, my brother called to tell me that my father had died suddenly of a heart attack.

In our culture, we put fresh rose petals around the dead person and there is always a strong sweet smell, just like I had smelled the night before in bed.

If I ever had a doubt about whether we have souls, it was erased forever.

I think about this event often, and marvel at my father's courage, understanding, faith, and acceptance. He knew that his time had come and he wanted to leave this world, living and dying, the way he wanted. He wanted to leave it without being dependent on others for care, and walking on his own, which he still did at the age of 84. I believe my father was able to achieve this by accepting death when its time had come.

It can be helpful for those of us who are left behind to think of the departed as having passed on to the next chapter in their lives. As I struggled with what had to be one of the saddest times in my life (apart from the death of my mother), my wife Jean gave me a framed poem to help me cope and accept the loss of my father. This poem, written by Mary Elizabeth Frye, hangs in my room.

> Don't stand at my grave and weep
> I am not there, I do not sleep.
> I am a thousand winds that blow,
> I am the diamond glints on snow.
> I am the sunlight on ripened grain,
> I am the gentle autumn rain.

> When you awaken in the morning's hush,
> I am the swifter uplifting rush.
> Of quiet birds in circled flight,
> I am the soft star that shines at night.
>
> Do not stand at my grave and cry
> I am not there, I did not die.

Perhaps, as we see the wonders of everyday life, those of us who are physicians and healers can learn to accept that death will eventually find us all. Once we embrace this acceptance within ourselves, we can be helpful to others who need us so dearly in their time of pain and sorrow.

Having had that conversation about death with my father left me with the clear priorities and goals of living that he desired for his dignified and good death. Now, over 20 years later, helping others at the end of life has become my passion.

My passion is to ease suffering and assist families during a time when others may turn away or are very uncomfortable and ill at ease, and often unwilling to talk about the final phase of life. This is something my father's wisdom has taught me. He taught by example, something many of us come to eventually realize about our parents. They are always teaching us one way or another.

3 | THE GIFT

Before modern medicine, a person got old, got sick, and died – or just got sick and died. **Now, dying is not that simple.** A majority of people are dying in hospitals or nursing homes, and before doing so, are likely kept alive by machines, medicines, and enduring aggressive therapies, including treatments for cancer and surgeries, or artificial tube feedings unable to enjoy food orally.

It is because of this new paradigm in medicine that it now falls upon palliative care physicians to help relieve the resulting burden. The busy acute care physician is focused on saving life, prolonging life, treating the symptom and disease. This is where palliative care comes in, with the perspective of the big picture and the ability to focus on what is important to patients in the time that remains. **This process of advance care planning allows patients to articulate their goals and drives the plan of care to determine what treatments to offer in order to achieve these goals.**

Thus, holding these difficult conversations is the *"gift"* that the palliative care team, consisting of physicians, nurses, social workers, nurse practitioners, chaplains, and more, offers to the patient, the family, the other healthcare providers, and all those who support that patient – with focus on all aspects of suffering: physical, emotional, psycho-social, and spiritual.

This work completed by the palliative care team becomes **a *gift* to other clinicians** who do not have the time or the expertise to engage in this difficult task. The team is very helpful in looking at the big picture, explaining all that must be understood by the patient and family in simple terms, having family meetings no matter how much time they require, following the patient on an ongoing basis, and offering multidisciplinary support that covers all aspects of suffering.

It is also a *gift* to the patient because, having had the talk about future goals, the remainder of his or her life will be lived in a manner that makes the most sense. Once the goals to be achieved are clear, the treatment plan can be made to support them. If the patient's goals cannot be achieved, non-beneficial treatments (those that do not help achieve the goals) can be stopped or not offered. The patient can be kept comfortable, live the last days the way that he/she wants and achieve a dignified death with no unnecessary, non-beneficial procedures or treatments.

Conversations about death and dying and advance care planning that clearly define one's important goals and wishes is a *gift* to one's family – probably one of the best gifts one can give to one's children and loved ones. The family can now be guided by these wishes if the capacity for decision-making is lost and one or more members of the family must make decisions at this emotional time.

They will not have to make these hard decisions for their loved one on their own in the future. Decisions can now be based on what is known to be important to the loved one. **This reduces the burden on the family.** Since plan of care is now based on the patient's voiced wishes, values, and goals, **the family can be at peace with the decisions**, knowing they are making the right decisions as well as honoring their loved ones' wishes.

When a patient's wishes are not known, **our helping the family make hard choices that alleviate suffering is a "*gift*" from us to the family, and from the family to the dying patient**. As stated by one of my patient's family members, the sister of a 53-year-old lady in the terminal stages of CP, "Letting our sister die in peace now is a gift from us to her."

LETTING GO IS A MAJOR ACT OF LOVE AND A GIFT

4 | DESCRIBING PALLIATIVE CARE AND HOSPICE CARE

The National Consensus Project for Quality Palliative Care describes palliative care in this way:

Palliative care means patient and family centered care that optimizes quality of life by anticipating, preventing, and treating suffering.

Palliative care throughout the continuum of illness involves addressing physical, intellectual, emotional, social, and spiritual needs and (facilitating) patient autonomy, access to information and choice.

Palliative Care.org describes palliative care as follows:

Palliative care is a specialized medical care for people with serious illness. It focuses on providing relief from symptoms and stress of a serious illness. The goal is to improve quality of life for both patient and family. It adds an extra layer of support.

It's never too late to lessen the burden. It improves QOL, provides close communication, and a partnership of palliative care team, patient, and family.

    1. As palliative care physicians, we provide additional, supportive service to help many aspects of a patient's care. Our multidisciplinary team of doctors, nurses, social workers, chaplains, and volunteers

helps with **all** symptom management, including pain, and we also help the patient and family deal with any psychosocial, emotional, and spiritual issues

2. We also help patients, their families, and their doctors in **goal-setting and advance care planning.** By helping establish goals of care, we can then, along with the primary physician, work on a plan of care which will help achieve these goals.

Our role is especially helpful with making difficult decisions for treatment choices, now or in the future. We help patients and those supporting them decide why a certain treatment may be advisable or not. **We help give reason to the decisions so they are not just based on emotion, and in the end help all be at peace that what was done was in the loved one's best interest.**

Palliative care can be delivered right alongside curative therapies.

Hospice care is the same multidisciplinary palliative care of patient and family that occurs during the last six months of adult life as a Medicare benefit. In children, many times it is provided concurrently with curative and acute services. Most of hospice care is delivered in the home, at a time when goals of care are mainly comfort only. Inpatient hospice care is available when symptoms are severe and cannot be managed in the home.

Explaining Palliative Care and Hospice to Patients

Most people, including patients, families, physicians (unless you are a palliative care physician, of course), and other health-care workers, do not quite understand what **palliative care** is, so saying, "I am a palliative care consultant" is not enough. Over the years I have come to explain what I do to patients and families in this way:

I am a palliative care physician. Let me explain what I do.

I add an additional layer of support in your care, and these palliative care services can be provided right along with curative treatments. Apart from helping with the management of different physical symptoms, including pain, I help the doctors, patients, and families with their decision-making for now and for the future. We call it advance care planning. I help you make choices that would be best for you the patient (or, if talking to family, your loved one), giving reasons why one treatment makes sense over the other. This way you will be at peace in the end, knowing that you are making the right decision, a decision based on reason and rationale and not just emotion alone.

The goal here is to make decisions that are in your best interest (or your loved one, if talking to family), keeping your (his or her) values and wishes foremost. I will help you do that. These are emotional times and it is difficult to make good rational decisions when one is emotionally upset. You would not go out to even, let's say, buy a car, or make any other big decision when emotionally upset.

These are huge decisions here. I am going to help you look at the big picture and help you understand why a certain decision would be better than the another, give you reasons for why it makes sense to do A versus B, **so you will be at peace that you are doing what is right for you (or your loved one)***. To do this well, I need to know you (your loved one) better, so tell me a little bit about yourself (her or him) – what you (he/she) did, how you (she or he) lived, what is important to you (him/her).* [In addition, if talking to a family member, ask if their loved one ever had any conversations about nearing end of life, and how he/she may have wished to live, or not.]

***You are (or,* if talking to a family member making decisions for a loved one,** *your loved one is) number one and decisions are to be made keeping your (your loved one's) "good" and "interest" prime*. *And I am here to help you to see why certain choices would be the right choices. Instead of getting stuck with specific treatments, we are going to concentrate on your goals, look at the big picture to see where we are headed and what that looks like, now and in the future. All decisions are primarily going to be made from the standpoint of what is most beneficial in achieving your goals.* [When talking to a family member, add: *Although you, the family, are very important, we have to keep remembering that the patient, your father/mother/etc., in this case, comes first. He/she is number one and you are a close second. All decisions to be made need to clearly be good for him/her.*]

I can also help clarify other medical conditions, treatments, test results, etc. that may be confusing to you. Our team of professionals (doctors, nurses, social workers, chaplains and volunteers) adds another layer of supportive care to help decrease the suffering by dealing with pain and other symptom management along with help for any psychosocial and spiritual issues."

Hopefully the role of the palliative care team becomes clearer to others when explained thus.

Since most public is leery of the "H" word when recommending **hospice care**, I usually just describe what it is first. The conversation may go something like this:

"Looks *like the goal now is mainly to keep you comfortable. How would you like if we were to send you home and arrange for support services so that you have a nurse, a social worker, a chaplain, and volunteers making regular visits to see that you are well cared for? Your physician is also a member of the team and can visit if necessary.*

We can manage the pain and other symptoms at home with a nurse who is available 24/7. A physician will be available by phone for any questions. You will not have to return to the hospital for managing symptoms. If you get worse, we can manage at home with the help of the team. Does this sound good to you?*

If the answer is in the affirmative, then we proceed to tell them:

Now, these services are under the umbrella of what is called hospice. The goal is to keep you as well as you can be for as long as possible during whatever time you have left.

If we cannot manage your illness at home, you can be sent to an in-patient unit of the hospice. The other team members

can be very helpful with any emotional, social, and spiritual issues you may have. How would this work for you?
If you are interested, we can have a hospice liaison come and see you very soon.

Note that we avoid using the name hospice until we have described the services provided and the family seems to be receptive. We want them to know first what hospice care is and not get frightened by the name alone.

5 | COMMUNICATION – THE KEY TO GOOD PALLIATIVE CARE, RESOLVING CONFLICT AND MISUNDERSTANDING

In any relationship conflict is inevitable, but combat is voluntary.

In the healthcare setting, at home, or in the hospital, multiple parties can be involved in clinical conflicts. These include patient and family members, physicians, nurses, social workers, residents, and students, attending staff, administration, and other healthcare workers.

Conflicts arise around:

- Information (incomplete or misinterpreted, inaccurate, conflicting, or from multiple sources)
- Values (cultural, religious, experiential)
- Emotional States (shock, anxiety, fear, anger, frustration, hopelessness, etc.)
- Decision-Making (lack of goal identification, burdening family with the task of making hard decisions on their own)
- Communication:
    - Relying on medical lingo
    - Evading telling the truth
    - Giving false hopes

- Playing the telephone-tag game (talking to one or a few persons who in turn relay information as they understand it to others)
- Fragmented case discussion among professionals
- Lack of timely case conferences with family
- Poor listening skills of professionals
- Inability to focus under stress
- Unavailability of physician to patient/family

- Physician Attitudes/Medical Culture:
  - Technology and *the miracle* of science
  - Inability to accept death
  - Death = failure
  - Fear of lawsuits
  - Lack of familiarity with law and ethics
  - Ignorance about palliative care and hospice care
  - Difficulty with being candid with painful news
  - Fear of diminishing hope
  - Unpredictability of outcomes
  - Focus on the disease and not the whole person

Ten Steps to Prevent Conflict Near End of Life:
1. **Appoint point persons**: family and healthcare professionals
2. *Identify* the decision-makers
3. *Build trust*: keep your word
4. Be *clear, candid, and kind* about the diagnosis, prognosis, and progress of the patient
5. Clarify the *goals* of treatment and *make* the hard decisions for the patients' good, **giving reasons why**
6. Explain and ask for reasons (**the why question**) for the requested proposed course of action
7. *Get second opinion or consultation early*
8. *Respect patient/family wishes and values* – make advance directives/*advance care planning* a routine for every patient
9. Develop effective *communication skills:*
    o *Listen while keeping an open mind.*
    o *Practice passive listening:* be mindful of your facial expression, lean forward, make eye contact, use gestures, nod, use short vocalizations like "Ah," "Umm," "Oh," "I see," etc.
    o *Practice active listening:* paraphrase; use reflective statements, especially of the feelings expressed, like "It sounds like a very difficult ordeal." "How frustrating." "What I am hearing is…"

- Use **open-ended statements and questions, such as** "Tell me more." "Tell me what you understand." "What do you think happened?"
- *After asking key questions, follow up with the* **why question**: it clarifies the reasons for feelings and choices. "Why is this problematic? How does this help achieve the goals? Why is this so important?"
- Use **"I" Messages.** Speak in terms of your perceptions, such as "When you talk about this I sense a lot of anger." "I feel you may want to say something more." "I feel frustrated when all the information is not on the table. Is it like that for you too?"
- **Summarize.** It's very important to make sure everybody is on the same page. Summarize what was discussed and agreed upon for now, as well as the future plan.
- **Clarify.** Ask questions to assure you clearly understood what was said and what was meant." So, you do not want aggressive treatments no matter what because you think...?" *Also ask others to tell you what they understand from what you have just said.*
- **Reframe.** Rephrase what you hear to make it more helpful to the discussion and resolving issues. For example, if the original message was "The staff here is no good. Nobody pays attention to detail," you could rephrase this as, "Continued poor response certainly is very

discouraging and frustrating. Let us see what further might help."
- o Be mindful of the body language. Be aware of yours and notice theirs. What are you saying and what do you read?
(Gibson and West, 1992)
10. Have case conferences with staff and family early and frequently....

If the above steps are followed diligently it can be very helpful in decreasing conflict and making it a lot more manageable early in the game.

Reference:

Mediation and Facilitation: Developing Communication Skills by Joan M Gibson and Mary Beth West 1992

*Time is a tool —
use as much of it as you can*

More time with patients and family, less with computers

6 | BASIC RULES FOR HAVING DIFFICULT CONVERSATIONS AND GIVING "BAD NEWS"

A lot is written and available from many sources on how to give "bad news" or have the difficult conversations, (Buckman 1992, 1998), such as the SPIKES six-point protocol (Baile, 2000)

The first thing to remember is that this conversation is not necessarily a one-time affair. As a matter of fact, **it is an ongoing process** that may take several sit-down sessions to complete. (Buckman, 1992, 1998)

Basic Rules and Guidelines:

1. **PLAN AND PREPARE**: Review chart, consult with others as necessary, have all the pertinent information at hand before the meeting.

2. **PICK THE TIME AND TIMING:** Be prepared to spend **as much time as necessary**. Clear your calendar, and pick a time that is convenient to all parties involved. You cannot be in a hurry. It is important for patients and families to feel that you are here for them, so sit down and take all the time that is necessary. In my experience, it takes about 45 minutes to an hour on average. My shortest family meeting was 20 minutes and the longest was 2 ½ hours. **Timing is**

important. **Having the right people there is important.** You may have to meet in the evening or over the weekend so that decisions are made in a timely fashion. On the other hand, delaying a meeting even by a day or two may be preferable if it means all the key players can be there.

3. **CHOOSE THE PLACE/SETTING: Sit down** in a quiet, comfortable private room if possible. Granted, you may have to meet in the patient's room. If so, pull up a chair and **be at eye level.** Maintain a therapeutic distance (Two to three feet between two people) and **lean in** as you converse. **Do not sit behind your desk.** Sitting in a circle is preferable. Have cups, water, drinks, tissues available to all.

4. **HOLD A FAMILY MEETING: For good communication to occur, there is no better tool than to have as many of the key family members and the key members of the healthcare team as possible around the table at the same time.**

    This way everyone hears the same information, and everyone can voice their opinions and have their questions answered. A family meeting done well is crucial to good decision-making. Talking to a son on the phone or a wife in the hallway is not a family meeting, where tough decisions and goals of care are carefully crafted. Have the right key people there.

    At the start of the meeting make sure **everyone from all sides gets introduced** with their **names** and **roles, and relationship** to the patient.

When talking to families, it is imperative that you **refer to their loved one by name or relation: your father, grandpa, Mom, Mr. Jones, Mrs. Smith, etc. and not as patient only.**

The role of the chairperson is key to a good meeting. The Chair sees that the meeting runs smoothly, ensures that **everyone is recognized and given a chance to say what they need to,** keeps interruptions down, maintains focus, and serves as an active listener.

This active listening allows him/her to **clarify and simplify** what is voiced and **assure that people have heard and understood what was said.** The Chair's job is to help guide the discussion so as to achieve a joint decision based on rational reasoning.

5. **ALLOW NO INTERRUPTIONS:** None. No cell phones or calls permitted.

6. **KEEP THE LANGUAGE SINCERE, SIMPLE, SHORT, AND SWEET. No medical lingo. Explain medical terms in simple language.** Do not assume everyone understands it all. Keep asking if they understand and if there are any questions. **Have them repeat what they understand so that communication is clear. Be factual but not overly optimistic or overly pessimistic.**

For example, explain what DNAR or NO CPR means and reassure that care will never stop. *"All treatments will continue as they are. But if, despite our efforts, the heart stops, we will not attempt to resuscitate – no pushing on chest or giving electric shocks. Instead we will let nature take its course and let the patient die naturally, in peace.*

Please be reassured that a DNAR order does not mean do not treat. Again, all treatments and care will continue as they are now until there is an arrest, such as the heart and breathing stopping; essentially, he/she dies. Then we will not resuscitate, but let him go in peace.

Do you understand? Do you have any questions about CPR?"

7. **CLOSE THE INFORMATION GAP:** Use the Ask-Tell-Ask model (UCSF 2014). In other words, find out what they know, how much they want to know, then tell them what they did not know, and ask again to tell you what they understand from what you just told them.

   ASK.

   First ask the patient/family what they understand about the diagnosis, prognosis, present situation, clinical progress, treatments, and their response and the facts of the given case. <u>Almost always, patients and family members do not have all the facts straight. And their understanding differs among themselves as to what the facts are.</u>

   It is paramount to have the families talk about the sick person's life first, so you may wish to start off with:

"It is hard to make decisions without knowing your father. So first tell me about him, his life, his likes and dislikes, and how he was functioning before he got sick this time and then what happened. Then tell me what you understand is going on with his illness, diagnosis, the treatments, prognosis, etc."
Let them talk and *you listen and listen*.
Next, ask how they wish to receive the information – in great detail or just the bottom line? This enables you to gear your answers to their wishes.

TELL.

Warning Shot: Before giving "bad news", it is advisable to give what is referred to as a warning shot. A warning shot is a lead-in statement that allows people to brace themselves and get ready to absorb what comes next. This can help to decrease the severity of the impending shock. *"I am afraid I do not have good news"* or *"This may come as a shock to you...."* are two examples.

Share Information: Next, **give the facts in simple, understandable, and caring language**, using the same general vocabulary as the patient/family. Avoid medical terms. If you must use some, explain what they mean.

"This is going to be so hard. We were hoping that the new treatments would have shrunk the tumor. Unfortunately, what the scans show is that the tumor is twice its size and has now spread out to the lungs. I am so sorry that medicines have not helped. We were

hoping for at least a halt in the spread. We are surprised and dismayed, as you must be."

Be clear with the diagnosis and prognosis. Be very clear as to what the diagnosis means and what can be expected in the future. Too often all the family knows is what treatments are being offered for the "problem" or the disease, without understanding the overall picture, such as chances of survival and the duration, clinical trend, severity of the illness, and quality of life.

Address pros and cons of suggested options and the quality of life issues.

As long as we keep offering new treatments, the message they are receiving is that we can "fix" this. If "it" cannot be fixed, then we are giving the wrong message by continuing to offer non-beneficial treatments.

ASK.

To ensure that you have communicated clearly, **ask the family/patient to tell you what they have understood and again correct any misinformation.**

Now you have "closed the information gap" and everybody is on the same page.

8. **ENGAGE IN THERAPEUTIC SILENCE:** When families/patients are very upset or quiet, be quiet yourself and give them time to "digest" this for a while. **Be quiet, but be present**, and stay with them, giving emotional support (not checking your phone messages).

9. **EMPATHIZE:** Empathy is paramount for good communication in the patient-physician relationship. It needs to be present as often and as much as needed throughout our interactions with patients and families.

Upon hearing the clear diagnosis/prognosis and the facts, there is an emotional reaction from the family or the patient. Your job is to empathize now, namely **acknowledge and validate the emotion and voice your understanding of the possible reasons for their reaction.**

The best initial response is to be quiet, **show caring presence**, let the emotion subside some, and let their body language show you that they are ready for input before acting. Families appreciate the physician just "being there."

We are not saying "I know how you feel," but noticing and acknowledging their emotions – sad, angry, disappointed, distressed, devastated, upset, surprised, etc. We are telling them that we see their emotion and we can see the reason why they might feel the way they DO.

"I *see you are very angry and distressed. It is understandable, because you never expected this since it looked like he was getting better. It is so hard when it is your child. I am sorry, and I wish I could give you better news, but I have to be honest about the facts. I wish things were different."*

"*You look so sad. This is very hard for you. It is never easy to realize you may lose your mother.*

Although we know one day we all have to go, but when the time comes it still is very painful. I wish life was easier in some way but this loss we all have to experience."

The family then sees that you notice their suffering and the reason for it and feels a little supported, understood. This helps build a connection between you and them.

This brings you a little closer to them.

In the realm of building relationships, being a good listener and having the skill to empathize are two major keys. Both can be learned and developed.

10. **TAKE TIME OUT:** If it is difficult to continue the conversation at this point, you can always opt to take a time out and regroup at a later time or another day.

    "Why don't we, if you wish, take some time off now and get together again later at a time of your choosing? Or would you rather continue? When would it be most convenient to you all? We will talk further then about any questions and decisions, goals and further plan of care..."

    Most of the time, patient and families are able to continue on. If so, talk about and clarify rational goals of care, which in turn will drive the plan of care.

11. **SUMMARIZE and PLAN for FOLLOW UP:** At the end of the meeting, summarize and clearly reiterate what is going to happen, what has been agreed upon concerning the goals of care and plan of care, who will

do what, what outcomes we are hoping for, and when to meet again for follow up next.

Write it all down, including what was discussed and next steps, along with your contact information and information on the next meeting, etc.

12. **THANK EVERYONE:** Thank everyone for attending, **shake hands, touch, hug as appropriate, and give out contact information**. Give out written instructions as appropriate and necessary.

    Document a brief summary of the meeting in the chart.

References:

1. Buckman R. How to Break Bad News: A Guide for Healthcare Professionals. Baltimore, MD: *Johns Hopkins University Press*, 1992
2. Buckman R. Communication in Palliative Care: a practical guide. In Doyle D, Hanks GWC, MacDonald N, eds. *Oxford Textbook of Palliative Medicine. 2nd ed.* New York, NY: Oxford University press; 1998:141 156
3. Baile, WF et al. SPIKES- a six-step protocol for delivering bad news: application to the patient with cancer. *Oncologist.* 2000:5(4):302-311.
4. University of California San Francisco Center for Excellence in Primary Care. Health coaching curriculum.

5. http://cepc.ucsf.edu/sites/cepc.ucsf.edu/files/Curriculum-sample-14-0602.pdf. Updated 2012

Recommended Resources:

- Vital Talk: vitaltalk.org
- Onco-Talk: depts.washington.edu/oncotalk
- AAHPM's Essentials Learning Module Five publication   on communication and teamwork
- Dr. Diane Meier's YouTube video, "The Human Connection of Palliative Care: Ten Steps for What to Say and Do" (one of my favorites)

7 | THE POWER OF TOUCH

Touch is a very powerful means of communication and valuable in reducing feelings of isolation. Use it appropriately at the right time. When appropriate, touch on the shoulder, arm or even a hug may be very appropriate, reassuring and comforting to the person. **Be very aware of and respectful of cultural differences.** Do not touch if the other party seems uncomfortable. Look for nonverbal language cues. If you are not sure, ask. *"May I give you a hug?"*

Be aware of **body language.** What are you saying by how you are behaving? What do you read in others?

Our job is not to keep people from dying no matter what, but to take care of them, decrease their suffering and help them heal even if they are dying so that they live and die as well as possible.

8 | THE POWER OF PRAYER

You may at times even wish to pray for the patient along with the family and colleagues. I would ask for permission to do so. *"Would it be ok if we together said a quiet prayer for your grandfather?"* It can be a silent prayer, so everyone can pray the way they wish according to their faith.

EVERYTHING THAT IS
OF BENEFIT
TO THE PATIENT
IS BEING DONE,
HAS BEEN DONE,
AND WILL BE DONE.
ONLY THE TREATMENTS
THAT ARE OF NO BENEFIT
WILL BE STOPPED
OR NOT OFFERED.

9 | REALISTIC HOPE

One detail that separates palliative care physicians from other specialties in medicine is that we are charged with giving our patients hope that is realistic without being defeatist.

What do I mean by that? Most of us are familiar with the saying, "Hope for the best and prepare of the worst." This attitude and way of being with patients may be ok in the early stages of a life-limiting illness. Yet as palliative care physicians we can do more.

We can help our patients to understand the true nature of their disease progression by beginning with, *"Realistically I would expect the following..."* and then perhaps ends with questions like:

> *What are you hoping for?*
> *What are your fears?*
> *What are your desired results?*
> *What is meaningful to you at a minimum?*

This later stage of disease management is often mistakenly thought to be the point when all are giving up hope, but I believe this type of thinking is quite misdirected. We must understand that hope during a terminal disease is not a linear progression from cure to death.

Hope changes as time and disease march on.

What begins as a hope for a mistaken diagnosis becomes the hope for a miracle from a second opinion. Then it becomes hope for a cure, then hope for another remission, then hope for a little more time, followed by hope for less pain, and finally hope to end suffering.

Hope for another year, month, week, day, or even an hour of "good" times spent together is hope that is worthwhile. I found this beautifully illustrated by the father of one of my patients.

His 16-year-old daughter was actively dying of brain cancer and was in a comatose state. During my home visit he confided in me that he hoped for just one more moment of looking in her eyes like he had done the day before. This father said, "You know, doc, yesterday she opened her eyes, so I just lay in the bed with her and gazed into her eyes for a good 45 minutes. That was the best day! Now I am just hoping for one more moment like that again."

10 | THE ETHICAL QUESTION FOR THE PHYSICIAN

If, as a physician, you are helping prolong someone's life by any artificial means, be it medicines (insulin, vasopressors, antibiotics, cardiac meds, steroids, thyroid meds, etc.) or machines (vents, dialysis, pacemakers, defibrillators, etc.) or artificial nutrition/hydration, the question before you is:

***Am I helping to prolong a meaningful life? OR
Am I just prolonging the dying, and increasing pain and suffering in the process?***

The suffering may also extend to the family and the caregivers.

If we knew the minimum levels of function that were acceptable to the patient with the help of life-prolonging treatments, then we would know when we were prolonging a meaningful life.

We cannot be sure of the good we are doing to patients if we do not know what is important to them.

How do we find that out? By asking. Talk to the patients about their wishes regarding the life they would want to live or not near the end. In other words, by doing the advance care planning (ACP) in a timely fashion while patients still have their capacity to make their own decisions. This can be accomplished with the help of "The Three Questions" as follows in the next chapters.

CARING PRESENCE and SILENCE CAN be VERY THERAPEUTIC

11 | ADVANCE CARE PLANNING FOR END OF LIFE (EOL) IN THE *INPATIENT* SETTING – "THE THREE QUESTIONS" TO ESTABLISH MINIMUM GOALS OF LIVING: A WAY TO SET MINIMUM THRESHOLDS FOR SUPPORTING LIFE BY ARTIFICIAL MEANS

Physicians face challenges every day. How to treat a patient is more problematic in the ICU setting if the goals to be achieved by various treatments have not been defined with the patient's input and periodically redefined. End of life decisions are easier when we have clearly established the minimum thresholds of living for every individual patient. So, to improve end of life care, healthcare workers first need to feel comfortable with accepting death as a normal natural part of life. (Aziz, 1996)

This makes it possible to have conversations with patients at an early opportune time ***while they still have capacity*** to make healthcare decisions, thus the choices made in the ICU reflect what the patient himself/ herself wanted.

This process of advance care planning is the key to decreasing suffering at the end of life for all concerned. (Emanuel, 1996; Messinger, 2009; Grossman, 2009).

If patients lose their capacity for making health care decisions without having expressed their desires, surrogate decision-making will be necessary.

Present day official state-sponsored advance directive documents, although helpful, are long (8-12 pages), narrow in scope, and difficult to understand by lay persons. They focus on death and dying, and many people have a hard time talking about such concepts.

This chapter presents a pragmatic guide for professionals when end of life decision-making discussions are taking place. It focuses on guiding the professional to enable the patient in determining his or her acceptable quality of life. It focuses on *how to live* with or without the help of various life-prolonging treatments as chosen by the patient himself.

The big question is whether or not we are supporting a meaningful life through life-prolonging treatments and procedure. When patients have clearly defined the level of physical and mental functioning that is meaningful to them, the healthcare team knows the goals to pursue.

There are many "life-prolonging artificial treatments" in the realm of medicines, machines and artificially provided nutrition and hydration, without which life could not be sustained by the patient himself or herself. Some examples would be: respirators, cardiac pacemakers or defibrillators, vasopressors, renal dialysis, and nutrition and/or hydration via tubes (N/G or PEG) or

IV. Also included are any and all other treatments, such as antibiotics, heart meds, insulin, or blood transfusions, if they are helping to maintain or prolong life.

Where, when, and how to have discussions with patients and family?

Ideally, such conversations ought to take place in physicians' offices before major illness strikes, as a part of routine well care and advance care planning for the future – or at least at the first signs of a major illness, especially a life-limiting illness like cancer, a stroke, heart, lung, or kidney failure, or any signs of neurologic decline or disease.

In the hospital setting, if this conversation has not yet been held, the attending, intern, or the resident ought to talk to the patient as soon as the opportunity arises – if the patient still has capacity to make healthcare decisions. Presence of family is preferred if the patient does not object, but it is not mandatory.

If the patient has lost capacity already, you are then forced to talk only to the family about goal setting. (See Chapter 17, "Helping Surrogates Make Decisions.") Another healthcare worker (MD, RN, social worker, etc.) needs to be in the room as a witness to your conversation. If time allows, it's best to schedule these discussions as goal setting meetings, with ample time allotted and sufficient space provided for all to comfortably sit down to talk. It's critical to keep precise notes. In a simplified manner the conversation revolves around the three basic questions to ascertain what is meaningful life for one (Stoddard 1996).

When speaking with a patient who has capacity, **The Three Questions are:**

1. What is the minimum level of *mental functioning* that is acceptable to you with the help of life-prolonging treatments?
2. What is the minimum level of *physical functioning* that is acceptable to you with the help of life-prolonging treatments?
3. What life-prolonging treatments are you willing to use or not (indefinitely or for a trial period) if they can get you to your minimum acceptable level of functioning?

<u>Suggested conversation with the hospitalized patient and family</u>:

One might say the following:

Our talk/discussion today is going to focus on setting goals for your treatment in order to achieve at least your minimum goals of living in three major areas of concern.

We can certainly discuss anything more that you may wish, and let me remind you that as long as you are able to make your own decisions, **you can always change your preferences at any time.** *None of this is etched in stone.*

These three areas are: one, your mental functioning or awareness; two, your physical state and function; and three, the use of artificial treatments and the length of time that you are willing to endure them.

As a physician, you always work off the baseline function of the patient. If you do not know the baseline, you do not know what goals are possible and where you are headed to.

So, you would say:

Before we get to The Three Questions, I would like to know you a little bit better. I would like to know how you were functioning before you got sick this time. In other words, what was your baseline function and how did you consider your quality of life to be?

(This gives us an idea of what we can hope for in the best-case scenario. Your recommendations as a physician may be different knowing how well or how poorly the patient was functioning at home. **You will also build a little bond by knowing your patient better and be able to guide him/her more rationally**.)

It's now time to ask Question One.

*Now, let's first talk about establishing minimum goals for **mental awareness**.*

Our hope, of course, is to at least get you back to functioning at the level that you were before you got sick this time.

But if you continue to worsen, what level of decreased mental function/awareness is still acceptable to you with help of life-prolonging treatment? Let me explain some of these treatments to you.

(Give examples of what is pertinent to that specific patient, whether it's a PEG tube, respirator, dialysis, pacemaker, cardiac meds, insulin, antibiotics, etc.)

To help you understand better and think, let me give you examples of some of the different levels of mental awareness.

- *Fully aware and having the capacity to make your own decisions*
- *Aware but unable to make your own decisions, but still able to converse well*
- *Able to recognize family and friends and can communicate verbally*
- *Able to recognize people and can communicate but not verbally*
- *Able to recognize family, can focus on TV, but cannot communicate*
- *Able to keep eyes open but unable to focus*
- *Totally unaware of surroundings and people*

Allow the patient to choose what level of functioning is acceptable and meaningful when he/she is on life-prolonging treatments.

It may even be easier to comprehend if you start from the lowest level of unconsciousness and go up.

Once the patient has decided, ask for the reasons for choosing this, then reiterate what the patient has said and have him/her reaffirm.

It's now time to ask Question Two, to establish minimum goals for physical abilities.

Let's now address the issue of physical capabilities. What level of physical functioning is acceptable to you with artificial life-prolonging treatments? Some scenarios may be as follows:

- *Mostly in bed, but able to get up and go to the bathroom by yourself, feed yourself, and are able to swallow*
- *Bedridden, can go to the bathroom only with assistance, but still able to feed yourself and swallow*
- *Bedridden and unable to go to the bathroom, must use a bedpan, but still able to feed self*
- *Bedridden, can go to the bathroom only with assistance and are unable to feed self, but still able to swallow.*
- *Incontinent, bedridden, need total care but able to swallow*
- *Cannot enjoy food, unable to feed orally, must be artificially fed by tubes or IV*

Obviously, there can be many other permutations to these. Major concerns patients seem to have are with mobility, the ability to get out of bed independently, ability to toilet and bathe, incontinence, talk, and the ability to swallow and enjoy food.

Once the patient decides what is acceptable and what is not, reiterate what he/she said, what it means and have them reaffirm.

Now it's time to address Question Three, use of artificial treatments.

Let's discuss treatments now. Are there any artificial treatments that you absolutely do not want, even for a short time? If so, what is your reason?

I choose what may be pertinent to that particular patient and explain in layman's terms (respirator with intubation, which is a tube inserted in the trachea through the mouth or nose, tracheostomy, which is a tube inserted directly into the trachea through a hole made surgically in the neck; artificial nutrition/hydration with tubes through the nose (N/G) or directly into the stomach (PEG) or through IVs, dialysis, etc.):

Mrs. Smith, since you are unable to swallow, it is possible to give you food and fluids through a tube surgically inserted directly into your stomach from the outside. It is called a PEG tube. We need to first discuss the benefits and possible complications of such a procedure...) and so on.

Important questions regarding life-prolonging treatments are:

- *Do you mind receiving some or any and all of these artificial treatments for a short period of time if we can at least get you to your minimum mental and physical function goals as we have just discussed?*
- *How many days would you say you are willing to try artificial treatments if there is no improvement?* ***You may also leave it up to the judgment of the physicians.*** *Once they are certain they cannot get you to your minimum acceptable levels, artificial treatments can be stopped in good faith. Your care will never stop, and all steps will be taken to assure you do not suffer.*
- *Do you have any specific questions about these or other treatments?*
- *Are there any treatments that you are absolutely against receiving? If so, why?*

Again, have the patient reaffirm what he/she said in reply to The Three Questions. Try to understand "why" in all the choices by asking patients their reasons for the decisions. If there are treatments the patient absolutely does not want, discuss their reasoning to assure they are not misguided.

Similarly, clarify myths and misconceptions about aggressive therapies like CPR, dialysis, and tube feedings. There is a place for aggressive treatments, so a "never put me on a machine" statement by a patient may be misguided. We need to ensure their reasons are based on facts, so we have to ask, inform, and truthfully guide.

While not in the case of terminal dementia, for example, there is a place for G tubes in the right scenarios, such as throat cancer while under treatment. This allows a patient to be nourished, and the feeding tube can be stopped once the patient is healed and able to swallow.

Patients may be refusing aggressive therapies under misconception. Patients might say "I never want to be on a vent!" not realizing that this could be lifesaving for a short duration while their infection or pulmonary embolism is being treated.

Open and full information is necessary for good informed decisions. The simplest way would be to ask the patient the reasons for his/her decisions. If the reasoning is based upon misinformation, it can be then corrected.

After you're clear that the patient's choices are based on accurate information, continue the conversation:

As long as we can achieve your minimum goals as discussed, we will continue to aggressively treat you as we are now.

Once it's clear that we cannot get you to your minimum goals, we will continue to manage your symptoms. We will ensure that you are comfortable, without pain and not suffering but all unnecessary and life-prolonging artificial treatments that are not helping us achieve your goals will be stopped.

Your care will always continue.

Regarding CPR Or NO CPR

I tend not to talk about No CPR or DNAR as such, but approach resuscitation in the following manner:

If, in spite of aggressive treatments, you have a cardiac or pulmonary arrest – in other words, your heart stops or you stop breathing – you will be resuscitated unless there is no chance of achieving your minimum goals of living as you have just defined. Is this okay with you?

Please understand that we will always continue to take good care of you and your care will never stop.

If the patient is already in a physical state where CPR would be medically or ethically wrong, then give patient/family reasons why it will not be done. (See Chapter 21, "Addressing DNR/DNAR.")

How your patient wants to die may also be addressed:

This may also be a good time to give some thought to how and where you may want to spend your last days when that time comes. Please talk to your family so that we and your family can honor your wishes.

Always summarize at the end:

Remember you can always change your preferences at any time you wish. Just let us know.

In summary, this is what you said as I understand it. (Repeat what the patient said.)

Here's an example:

This is what I heard you say:
1. *You do not want your life prolonged by artificial means:*
    - *Once you lose abilities to communicate, or*
    - *are totally bedridden, or*
    - *have been on respirator for 7 days with no improvement.*
2. *You do not want artificial tube feedings of any sort and no IV hydration either if it is not helping improve your status to the minimum level you have established.*
3. *You want to die at home with family and friends.*
4. *You wish to donate your body to science.*

In the end, always thank the patient and all of the family members who are there, then shake hands and ask if they have any questions. Be sincere and tell the patient something like this:

Now that you have shared what is important to you with us, we can take better care of you according to your wishes. I know this has been hard, but I want to thank you for sharing your thoughts and your time.

And you have just given a great gift to your family, *who will not have to struggle with decisions for you in case you are unable to do so yourself in the future. We are available any time you need us. You can reach us through your nurse or through this phone number.*

Also thank all others from the healthcare team who may be in the room. Additional words of caring are always welcome. Remember, we may not be able to cure always, but we can always care.

Documentation

It's very important to document these conversations, for the sake of all involved, including you. Here's what to do:

- Make a notation in the chart under "End of Life Discussions – Wishes and goals of treatment for Mr./Ms. X"
- List all who were present at discussion.
- Write the minimum goals of living as the patient has defined them, and any and all pertinent wishes.
- Sign your note.
- Have one of the witnesses from the healthcare team sign it too. Have it noted in the progress notes and keep a copy in the patient's chart. **This is now a legal document, essentially an oral advance directive in Maryland (please check your state laws)**
- Give a copy to patient and family and the attending physician.
- If the family was not present at discussions, talk to them personally and give a copy of the oral advance directive/patient's wishes.

Cases Studies

Here are three case studies to illustrate how much difference knowing a patient's minimum goals of living makes to patients, their families, and their healthcare providers.

Case # 1 – "This Sucks!"

The first case had no ACP and no directives when she was admitted to the ICU because of septic shock.

Beth is a 70-year-old lady who was diagnosed six months earlier with pancreatic adenocarcinoma with involvement of liver and gall bladder. She was presently receiving "palliative chemo."

Three months prior, she had small bowel obstruction and now has a G-tube to help with drainage. No surgery was possible. She has been maintained on TPN for these three months. Now, in the ICU, she is a full code, fully aware, with normal blood pressure, not requiring vasopressors to help keep blood pressure up, on IV antibiotics and nasal oxygen.

Luckily, when I saw her, she had decision-making capacity. I met with her and her two adult children.

We talked about the quality of life, The Three Questions, and her goals of living. She said her life now sucks. Her goals were to have mental and physical comfort. She did not want her life prolonged by any means if, at a minimum, she cannot recognize and communicate with her children. Physical restrictions did not matter as long as she could talk to her children. She did not want aggressive treatments anymore, but wanted the TPN to continue for now.

On the basis of the above we were able to advise her why a DNAR would make sense since, even if resuscitated, she would only be worse clinically. Giving treatments that would worsen her already poor quality of life would not be ethically right. She understood and agreed, as did the children.

Based on her goals of comfort and wish to be able to talk to her children, the following plan of care was formulated with her and family's ongoing input and agreement. She was reminded that any of this could be changed if she changed her mind anytime.

1. DNAR/DNI. Ok to use bag ventilation if needed.
2. Refer to hospice.
3. No blood transfusions.
4. Lab tests only to help with comfort care.
5. No return to hospital. Admit to in-patient hospice unit if unable to manage symptoms at home.
6. Oral antibiotics only to help with comfort.
7. TPN to continue until she cannot recognize or communicate with her children.
8. No dialysis.

A MOLST (Medical Orders for Life-Sustaining Treatments) form was filled and signed, and copies were given to patient and family.

As you can see, **The Three Questions help in reaching the minimum goals, which then help us with the plan of care. In other words, the goals of care drive the plan of care.**

Case # 2 – "The Retired Marine"

The second case had an advance directive based on The Three Questions.

This patient was a 92-year-old retired marine. He had been gradually losing weight and becoming more and more frail over the last nine months. After a loss of 50 pounds, he weighed just 110 pounds.

There is no major life-threatening illness present, although he is on some heart medications and pain pills for his back. Mentally he is sharp and has capacity to make his health care decisions. Physically he is very weak, lies in bed mostly, but is able to go to the bathroom himself and gets out of bed to eat.

One day he bumped his leg, which resulted in a hematoma above the ankle, which got infected, causing him to be hospitalized with fever. Gangrene and sepsis developed, which left him semiconscious and unable to decide.

Physicians recommended below knee amputation as the only recourse to saving his life and asked his wife for consent.

The wife then consulted with the author to help in the decision-making. We reviewed his answers to The Three Questions on his minimum goals of living and end of life wishes. Luckily, his advance directive was formulated two months earlier, at his last visit.

His end of life wishes and living plan were as follows:

1. Do not artificially prolong my life if I cannot recognize my family AND communicate with them.
2. You may treat my illness if I am able to recognize and communicate with my family but DO NOT artificially prolong this state by means of dialysis, respirator or artificial nutrition and hydration for more than a week.
3. If I am totally bedridden, please DO NOT treat any illness but keep me comfortable.
4. Artificial treatments are only acceptable if I can be rehabilitated to my goal as mentioned in # 2 above.
5. I do not want to be a burden to my family, and I want to die at home.

Since amputation would have certainly made him bedridden, a situation he did not want to live with as mentioned in # 3 above, and, given his frail and septic status, there was no chance of rehabilitating him with a prosthesis to the point where he could be ambulatory, it was decided not to amputate. He died two days later. The wife was at peace with her decision since she had his "goals of living" clearly defined in front of her and knew she was doing what he wanted. She was grateful for having established these goals just two months earlier. (She had her own advance directive done as well.)

Advance care planning is the key to easing the distress and suffering at the end of life

Case # 3 – "The Physician with a Checklist"

Compare the above experience to the one that Josh went through. Josh was a physician, an ophthalmologist by profession, and had **a "checklist" type advance directive which indicated that he did not want his life extended IF he was in a vegetative state. It did not mention any "goals**

of living" to indicate what was meaningful to him as far as living goes. He got ill and experienced multiple strokes.

Josh had a cardiac arrest and was resuscitated. His cognitive and physical function decreased slowly to the point where he was on a chronic vent with trach tube, unable to eat (PEG tube placed), and unable to smile or interact, but his eyes were open and he took a few breaths on his own.

Since he was not in a persistent vegetative state yet, his wife insisted on continuing the artificial treatments to honor his wishes. He lasted in this poor state for over six weeks before succumbing to sepsis. If we had had *goals of living* conversations with him instead of just a checklist, perhaps the end could have been more meaningful to him.

Can you see the importance of concentrating on goal-setting and on supporting living meaningfully?

Case # 4 – "Unwanted Treatments"

The fourth case is that of a 67-year-old lady with lung cancer who was very clear on what artificial treatments she did or did not want to live with and for how long.

The surgeons had recommended lobectomy but had warned her of the possibility of a respirator-assisted lifetime; however, she had the option to stop artificially life-prolonging treatments at any time.

The patient, again having full capacity, was able to voice very clearly that she did not want to live hooked to a respirator for life. She did agree to one week of ventilator support, but if she was unable to be weaned, she wanted the respirator stopped anyway. She wished to die rather than live hooked to a respirator.

In this case, she voiced her wishes in front of the doctors, her family, and the ethics committee as well.

After surgery, she could not be weaned successfully. The surgeon initially was very reluctant at seven days to have the ventilator stopped. **Because we had had a clear conversation with her about her choices and her reasons, however, we were able to help her achieve what she wished.** After ten days, the respirator was disconnected and she died. Pain, anxiety, and air hunger were well managed with medication.

Once again, knowing a patient's goals of living made decisions easier and easily acceptable to the family and health care team, since they were "her" decisions and not necessarily the physician's or the family's.

Also, the family did not have to struggle with making this very tough decision.

All these cases illustrate the simplicity of the document (only one page long), the clarity of instructions, and the relative ease of decision-making when the patient's goals of living are clearly known. The four cases also emphasize the need to have these discussions with patients early, while they still have capacity and are relatively well. **Thus, we can see that** these discussions need to happen with our patients soon, preferably *now*.

In addition, we all ought to have these discussions with our friends and loved ones about ourselves in a timely fashion. It will prevent heartache later.

Plus, by experiencing it yourself you will understand why sometimes it is hard for others to talk about this, and you will be able to help them better.

Even in situations where patients may not know what they want, a discussion like this will open the door for reflection and further future conversations. This may then lead to a more fruitful talks and goal-setting at a later time.

It is imperative that physicians be supportive and not unduly paternalistic in their approach. Knowing that the decisions of patients, and the resulting plans, are not etched in stone and that choices can be changed anytime as one's thinking changes will allay any anxiety of being "stuck" with what one may choose today.

References:

1. Stoddard, Jim. 1998. "A Practical Approach to DNR Discussions" *Bioethics Forum* 14(1):27-32
2. Messinger - Rapport, BJ. Advance Care Planning: beyond the living will. *CCJM*.2009;76(5)276-285
3. Grossman, D. Advance care planning is an art not an algorithm. *CCJM*.2009;76(5):287-288
4. Emanuel LL, Danis M, Pearlman RA, Singer PA. Advance care planning as a process: structuring

the discussions in practice. *J Am Geriatric Soc.* 1995.43(4):440-446
5. Aziz, S. Accepting Death. *HEC FORUM.* 1996; 8(2): 126-132

12 | ADVANCE CARE PLANNING FOR END OF LIFE (EOL) AND "THE THREE QUESTIONS" IN THE *OUTPATIENT* SETTING

Advance Care Planning (ACP) is a process that is essential for adults at any age regardless of their state of health, whether they are well or ill. It helps them understand and share with family and healthcare givers their personal values, life goals, wishes, and preferences regarding future quality of life and medical care.

ACP may include completion of an advance directive, which can include a living will indicating treatment choices near end of life and a durable power of attorney designation for healthcare decisions (DPAHC). The intent of ACP is to see that patients receive treatments and care that is in accordance with their goals, values, and beliefs.

ACP is an essential component of anticipatory guidance, which is the physician's responsibility. It is no different than advising about other health issues like nutrition, weight control, cholesterol, smoking, drinking, drugs, accident prevention, etc. **But are we, the physicians missing the boat when it comes to advance care planning**?

The low rates of advance directives (30%) in admitted patients, in my experience, (on the floors, in the ICU, or on the chronic vent unit) is an indication of the poor job we are doing in advising patients regarding end of life issues.

ACP is not getting done in a timely fashion on the sick patients, even after hospital admissions. **And if a patient does have a DNAR, this does not mean he/she has done advance care planning.**

I am now a believer that all hospital patients who do not have advance directives need to have their ACP done before they leave the hospital. **At a minimum, all patients with chronic illnesses, life-limiting illnesses, and dementia, as well as all ICU patients, need an automatic palliative care team consultation.**

Where I work, we are beginning the process of achieving ACP before patients are released. It is a tall order, so we will start with the healthcare workers, ethics committee members (got to practice what we preach), and the ICU, and expand as logistically feasible. No question it is the right goal to shoot for. Getting there will take effort and commitment.

I give six seminars yearly to the public on ACP at Chautauqua Institution in New York, where I lecture to about a hundred folks at a time.

When I ask how many of them have had their physician initiate discussions on end of life choices with them, sometimes no hands go up. And, at best, only 5-10% of the participants raise their hands.

This tells me that we are missing opportunities for anticipatory guidance about ACP in at least 90% or more of our patients.

Research has shown, and patients agree, that ACP can improve multiple outcomes, especially in patients with serious illnesses.

These benefits are as follows:
- Improved quality and length of life in patients with malignancies as well. Patients want their physicians to talk to them about their goals and have these discussions early. (Gesme, 2011)
- Increased rates of completion of advance directives. It also reduces stress, anxiety, and depression in the surviving relatives. (Detering, 2010)
- Reduction in hospitalizations at end of life (Teno, 2007)
- Increased likelihood that patient will die in their preferred place
- Increased use of hospice services

The Centers for Medicare & Medicaid Services (CMS) have now established billing codes for ACP. They are 99497 and 99498. CMS pays for ACP as a separate charge. You can also bill for Social Worker doing ACP under a physician's oversight as an "incident to" billing. (Jones, 2016)

There are so many opportunities to do advance care planning:
- At the yearly wellness exam
- At the first sign of any illness
- During a hospital admission for anything
- At first diagnosis of a life-limiting illness

- Year after year during the care of that life-limiting illness
- With clinical change in a patient with a chronic illness
- At hospital admission of a life-limiting illness
- At the first diagnosis and during management of cancer – it is really sad and disheartening to see patients with multiple years of cancer treatments, now with metastases in their last stages, who have had no conversations at all about end of life goals.
- At first signs of dementia – another very sad illness with patients suffering through a variety of issues just because we never advised and talked to them in a timely fashion.

Advanced care planning is a difficult subject to talk about with one's parents, children, or other loved ones, so most of us just avoid it. And, as physicians, we also avoid talking to our patients, most of us being just as uncomfortable. This is where courage is cultivated.

The problem is that meaningful life and living has a different connotation for everyone, and if we don't ask – and say for ourselves – then our last days of life may go very differently than we would wish.

Unfortunately, many times we only just *think* about the things that are important but never quite get around to *doing* them in earnest. Most of the time, life works out just fine despite our casual attitudes; however, we should be concerned with the possible "what ifs" that surface when these preferences are in reference to the quality of life we may have to endure if we, when the time comes, cannot speak for ourselves. **Without making a clear distinction, in writing or by conversation, we take the risk of living in a manner that we would not call a meaningful life – but may be powerless to change.**

Imagine that you have lost the capacity to make your own decisions and had never taken the opportunity to have end of life conversations with anyone. Your family is now left to complete this task for you. They must come to a consensus on "what they *think* you would have wanted." This is a heavy burden for a family to carry and one that could be avoided "if only" you had gotten around to it.

We owe it to ourselves and our families to have our EOL conversations with our loved ones, and as physicians, we owe it to our patients to address their end of life living goals by means of advance care planning in a timely fashion, while they still have decision-making capacity.

But when is a good time to do this?

The time to dialogue is now, while your patients have their wits about them, whether they have a serious illness or not. As physicians it is our responsibility to help establish clear goals of care which will then guide the plan of care for the patient.

The goal is to maintain the patient at the minimum acceptable level of functioning or better. Finding out what the patient envisions that life to be can be achieved by asking "The Three Questions" below.

To patients in outpatient settings who are in fairly good health and do not have a life-limiting illness, I may start this important dialogue by saying something like this:

"You are doing very well presently. But we are going to address a very important issue of planning for the future, how you would prefer to live near the end of life.

We do this with all patients now as a part of anticipatory guidance for issues we know may arise some day; when? no one knows. I myself had these talks with my family over 15 years ago.

The reason for talking now is that you have the wherewithal to know what is going on and can make your own decisions. God forbid if you were to lose that capacity, which can happen anytime to any one of us, before you made these decisions and shared them. Then your family would be left to make health care decisions for you. That is a big order. It would be good for them to know what is important to you.

Let's say at some time from now, if you get ill and your life is being prolonged by means of medicines or machines, that the level of your existence is meaningful to you. Then it is wonderful. But if the treatments are keeping you alive, but at a level lower than what you would consider meaningful, then it is of no good use and is only delaying the inevitable – and in the process making your life more painful and increasing suffering for you, your family, and friends.

So, you see, if we could establish that minimum level of meaningful existence for you, the doctors and hospitals would know when aggressive treatments are not warranted

and when just keeping you comfortable would be the best thing to do – just as you have chosen. Let's talk about that. It may sound complicated, but it's not. This can be accomplished by simply answering the following Three Questions to establish what kind of a life is worth living for you.

(NOTE: This is the same process detailed in the previous chapter for hospitalized patients, so you can refer to that for more details.)

1. *What is the minimum level of mental functioning (mental awareness level) that is acceptable to you with the help of life-prolonging treatments, whether they be medicines, machines, or artificially provided food and water via tubes or IVs?*
2. *What is the minimum level of physical functioning that is acceptable to you with the help of life-prolonging treatments?*
3. *What, if any, life-prolonging treatments are acceptable to you, or acceptable for a period of time to see if we can get you to your minimum acceptable level of function? Are there any known treatments you are opposed to and why?*

Our job as physicians is to guide. You may have to give examples of what lower levels of function may look like (as described in the previous chapter). **Most areas of concern for everyone have to do with independence, mobility, ability to bathe, toilet, eat and communicate.**

These three simple questions can help patients achieve more control at the end of life, even when they have lost the ability to make their own healthcare decisions.

These questions are basically the same whether the patient is relatively well or ill. The details of types of therapies may change some. All you are trying to do is establish the minimum goals when life is being prolonged artificially by some medicines or machines or artificial nutrition/hydration.

It is essential here to talk about goals to be achieved by whatever means are necessary rather than getting hooked on certain treatments, since it may not be clear earlier on in an illness – or before there even is an illness – as to what would be helpful.

My advice usually is that we give artificial treatments as long as there is a good chance that we can get the patient to their minimum acceptable levels of living as described by them. If we cannot achieve that, then artificial treatments would be stopped. The same is true of CPR – it is given if good chance of it being beneficial.

Now, if patients put their answers to The Three Questions in writing, give a copy to their family and physician, or even have a clear conversation with their family and physician, then hopefully they can be treated as they have wished. **Having one's wishes known to the family will be the best gift one can give one's loved ones.** Making one's own decisions so family will not have the burden of making these hard choices *is the gift*.

Unfortunately, there is no guarantee even then. Many times, the document is missing, cannot be located, or the family refuses to bring it. I had a patient's brother carry it around in his pocket for days before he finally was comfortable enough to share it with me.

This brings us to the importance of a **POA, power of attorney for healthcare decisions**, who is designated by the patient – someone who is agreeable, can be trusted to follow the patient's wishes, and can support patient's goals. (This person is not necessarily a close relative.)

Impress upon patients the need for dialogue with their POA so he/she understands where they are coming from and has the assurance that he/she can support them in achieving their goals at the end of life.

Examples

Here are some examples to illustrate how knowing – or not knowing – a patient's minimum goals of living has affected their families.

Example # 1 – "You Are the Experts"

Jonathan was 74-year-old in terminal stages of severe anoxic encephalopathy. The only family decision-maker was a 23-year-old nephew who was clearly struggling with the decision to limit and stop life-sustaining treatments. He finally said to the ethics committee members who were consulting, "Why don't you all make the decision instead of asking us? You are the experts!"

If Jonathan had had a conversation with his doctor or family members while he had capacity for decision-making, the burden would have certainly been reduced.

This also illustrates that, most of the time, the family is expecting us to make the big decisions, or at least guide the family instead of asking them what course of action to take.

Example # 2 – "The Father's Anguish"

Elena was 46, in the end stage of AIDS and on life support. Her father was a minister. While discussing the right course of action and contemplating quality of life and next steps, he said, "I know that I would not want to live like this myself. But she is my daughter. How can I stop life-sustaining treatments? We never talked about this happening."

Although Elena is very young, her illness demands of her physicians that they have the hard conversations of advance care planning, just in case. If those conversations had happened, it is probable that decisions would have been easier and burden on her father lessened.

I believe that it is up to us, the physicians, to bring up and pursue the questions of death and dying with patients, and their wishes on how to live, or not, at the end of life.

If patients, especially those who are older, and/or who have chronic and life-limiting illnesses, do not have any form of advance directive, living will, end of life living plan, five wishes, etc. and have had no end of life conversations; then I believe *we have failed in our mission of helping, healing and decreasing suffering*. We cannot just hope and wish that patients will do it on their own. We have to keep reminding and guiding them.

Example # 3 – "Thirty Years of Suffering"

My wife and I were travelling in the beautiful town of San Miguel Allende in Mexico and were on a city bus tour. Next to me sat a gentleman from the US, and in chatting about life and careers, I told him about my hospice and palliative care work and what it entailed.

After the two-hour tour, we all got out of the bus. He kept waiting for all to alight before he finally got out and said he wished to talk to me. He asked, "In your work that you do, you must have had to decide or help families decide and then stop life-sustaining treatments?"

"Oh yes, this comes up all the time," I said.

"Then how do you do it and what do you say? You see I had to decide about stopping life support on my wife 30 years ago after she had been in a car accident. And to this day I wonder if I did the right thing."

We had a long discussion then and I reaffirmed that he did do the right thing, since nothing good and meaningful could come out of continued life support after weeks of trial.

Letting his wife go was a big act of love, not to force her to suffer for his sake. Although it was sad and hard, it was the right thing for her. Prolonging a meaningless existence cannot be ethically justified. He had definitely done the right thing, I emphasized, a caring act for someone he loved dearly.

His eyes teared up, as did mine, and we hugged. He thanked me profusely and said, "You know, this has troubled me for 30 years. Thank you for helping me see that it was right."

Wow. What a burden he has carried for so long, even when he had made the right choice. **This again affirmed my belief that any little thing we can do to take the burden off the shoulders of the family is a gift to them.**

Even when they make the decisions, we need to affirm that their decision is right. Use kind, caring, supporting words and explanations so they will be at peace with it.

References:

1. Detering KM et al. The impact of advance care planning on end of life care in elderly patients: Randomized controlled trial *BMJ 2010;*340:c1345, Crossref. Medline
2. Gesme DH, Weisman M: Advance care planning with your patients. *J Oncol Pract 2011:* 7:e42-e44

3. Teno JM et al. Association between advance directives and end of life care: a national study. *J of Am Geriatr Soc.* 2007;55:189
4. Jones et al: Top 10 Tips in Advance Care Planning Codes in Palliative Medicine and Beyond, *J of Palliative Medicine*, doi:10.1089/jpm.2016.0202. e

*We don't just treat
a "disease" –
We render care to
a Person,
Manage their Illness,
Allay the Suffering
And support the Soul.*

13 | CREATING A DOCUMENT OF ACP/ADVANCE DIRECTIVE

There are numerous ways to create an ACP document or Advance Directive. One may use any of the pre-printed Advance Directive forms from their respective state (this includes living will and durable power of attorney for healthcare decisions) or other forms (such as The Five Wishes or the End of Life Living Goals and Plans as in this book's appendix). Although not necessary, many patients do elect to have a lawyer draw up these documents as a living will and a DPACH (durable power of attorney for healthcare decisions). Again, please check your state laws so you may advise patients correctly. One can also create one's own. This could even be handwritten, I suppose, but a typed document is preferable.

All wishes can be put in writing following the principles discussed earlier. These can include designation of a healthcare proxy (POA), what is important in life, instructions on treatment choices and any additional wishes regarding death and dying or living – where one wishes to die, organ donation, etc. (See the following chapter on "Examples of EOL Wishes and Living Plans.")

This document is then signed and witnessed by two persons. Under Maryland law neither witness can be the power of attorney for healthcare, and at least one of them must not be inheriting anything from the patient. Please know your local laws. Because of the different medical care implications, *strongly recommend to patients that when contemplating making advance directives, input from a physician, a nurse, nurse practitioner or a social worker familiar with EOL issues be sought.* In many states advance directives are not required to be done by a lawyer, or even notarized. Please check regulation and laws of the state you are in. Presently notarization is required in the states of Missouri, North Carolina, South Carolina, and West Virginia. This may of course change in time. My advice to patients is that even if you have a formal advance directive, add your minimum acceptable levels to it based on The Three Questions discussed earlier. Adding one's own thoughts and wishes in one's own words that spell out goals of living will make the document even better and more complete.

This now is a legal advance directive (check state/country laws) and is to be followed in case of illness.

Advise patients to be sure to give a copy to the POA for healthcare decisions, the family, doctors, lawyers and take a copy to hospital whenever they go there. Make it easily accessible, not locked in a safe deposit box as a patient of mine so proudly announced. **Even more important for the patients is to have had a discussion regarding their wishes and goals with the important people in their life (family, POA, and their physician, at a minimum).**

Carry a card in your wallet indicating that you have an advance directive/EOL living plan. Include the name of your physician, important members of your family, and the POA, and how to contact them.

Apart from the official state published advance directive forms, you may want to become familiar with some of the other **decision aids for advance care planning** that are available on the internet.

Here are some:

- **My Directives** (online tool at mydirectives.com)
- **Five Wishes** (Aging with Dignity)
- Consumer's Toolkit for Healthcare Advance Planning (American Bar Association)
- End-of-Life Decisions (Caring Connections, NHPCO)
- Conversation Starter Kit and how to talk to your doctor (The Conversation project)
- Tool kit at Compassion and Choices (Butler, 2014)

Sicker patients who are on restricted treatments (no CPR, no transfusions or dialysis, no artificial feedings, etc.) need a **MOLST** (Medical Orders for Life-Sustaining Treatments)/**POLST** (Physician Orders for Life-Sustaining Treatments) **or equivalent state approved form** filled and signed by a physician. Some states may have approved signed bracelets or electronic apps. **Know what is appropriate in the state you live in.**

Most patients who are a DNAR or have any other restricted treatment options have to have a hard copy of the POLST or other approved form readily available to healthcare workers and EMS so that they get cared for as they wish.

Without it, EMS personnel are obligated to use aggressive resuscitative measures.

Keep reminding patients to talk to their families and to their POA. **(First, or course, they need to ask someone if he/she is willing to be a POA and support them in their wishes and goals. And, second, they need to be forthcoming with their POA.)** My neighbor's 91-year-old mother flat-out refused to tell him what was in the living will that she had, saying, "It's none of your business!"

(We clearly have a lot of public education to do yet.)

Organ and Tissue Donation

Another one of our responsibilities is to remind patients to think about and if possible become donors and add that provision in their advance directives.

Reference:

M Butler et al "Decision aids for Advance Care Planning: An overview of the state of the science" *Ann Intern Med* 2014;161:408-41

14 | EXAMPLES OF END OF LIFE LIVING GOALS AND PLANS

Here are real life examples of EOL goals, wishes and plans from some of my patients. These are based on answers to The Three Questions to establish minimum acceptable levels of existence where life would still have meaning to the person, even though life is being prolonged with the help of some medicines or machines. (Names and some minor details are changed for privacy and confidentiality reasons.)

This shows how simple, easily understandable this process can be.

EXAMPLE #1: End of Life Goals for Mrs. JJ

JJ was 78 years old, with a long history of diabetes and COPD, now complicated by repeated hospitalizations over the last two years, along with heart failure. She was on continuous oxygen at home, able to get around with difficulty. She still had her capacity and enjoyed her meals. Her EOL wishes and living goals were as follows:

1. I do not want my life prolonged by any means if I am unable to communicate with my family (verbally or by gestures) even though I may be able to recognize them.

2. If I cannot get out of bed myself, please let me die in peace, do not extend my life by artificial medicines and machines.
3. Always make sure I am pain free and not suffering.
4. I do not want to be resuscitated if my heart or breathing stops.
5. I do not want to be tube fed if I cannot enjoy food by mouth.

signed by JJ and witnessed by two not closely related

Example # 2: End of Life Living Plan for MB

At the time of this conversation, MB had full capacity and was sitting in hospital bed doing crossword puzzles. We talked about planning for the future and asked her, if she worsens, what were her minimum acceptable levels of functioning to be supported by life-prolonging treatments?

She said, "I do not want my life prolonged by life-prolonging treatments if:

1. I am unable to communicate with my family. Or
2. I am totally bedbound and cannot get up even with help." Or
3. Unable to swallow food and drink.

This was documented in the progress notes and the note signed by me, the physician, and a nurse who witnessed the conversation. This is now essentially an oral advance directive. A copy was made to give to patient and family.

Although her directive was short, it was clear and helpful for the future planning of her care.

Example # 3: EOL Living Plan for WB

We talked with WB in the hospital in the presence of his two daughters and his nurse. He was 86 years old and had congestive heart failure, pneumonia with COPD. He had capacity and his wishes were as follows:

1. I do not want life prolonged by any means if I cannot recognize AND communicate with my family.
2. I also wish to receive no curative treatments if I am totally bed bound OR unable to eat and swallow.
3. I am willing for short term intubation if it can help me achieve the level of life as described above in #1.
4. I do not want to be resuscitated if I have a cardiac arrest now.
5. Dialysis and other treatments are OK only if it will help me to achieve mental awareness level as described in #1 and physically not be totally bed bound.
6. I want only comfort measures once it is clear that the minimum levels cannot be achieved as in #1 and #2 above.
7. I wish to die at home whenever that time comes.

Again, this was documented in his chart and signed by myself, the physician, and a witness, the nurse. This is now a legal document, an oral advance directive.

Copies were made and given to the family.

You can see from the above examples what a simple way this is to control your destiny. Most of the time this is not even a very long, time-consuming process as long as patients have decision-making capacity and are voicing their own choices.

It is when you have to talk to families and there are no directives from the patient that it becomes a time-consuming and difficult endeavor.

15 | PREPARING FOR DEMENTIA – THE SLOW DOWNWARD SPIRAL

In my experience of lecturing to thousands of people, one of the most fearful future situations that is always brought up is dementia, and how to approach the advance directives in a way that one suffers the least. Lay persons actually often openly ask if there is a way for them to end their life early if they get dementia. My advice when talking to patients is:

"At the earliest signs of dementia, please make your end of life living goals known, while you still have the capacity to make decisions. First know a little bit about the different stages of dementia and what to expect."

I acquaint them with the simplified version of the **Functional Assessment Staging Tool (FAST)** and its seven stages of the functional milestones in dementia:

Stage 1 – Normal adult with no cognitive loss.
Stage 2 – Normal adult with mild memory loss. **Subjective word finding difficulties.**
Stage 3 – Early Dementia: memory loss apparent to co-workers and family, such as being unable to remember the names of persons just introduced. **Decreased organizational capacity**.
Stage 4 – Mild or Early Stage Dementia: **decreased ability for complex tasks** like handling personal

finances and planning dinner for guests; decreasing memory of recent events.

Stage 5 – Moderate Dementia: **requires assistance in choosing proper clothing** for the day, occasion, or season.

Stage 6 a-e – Moderately Severe Dementia: Forgetting names of family. **Needing assistance with ADLs** (activities of daily living) such as toileting, bathing, dressing, and eating. May develop delusions, hallucinations, and obsessions. Anxiety and violence may develop. Start of incontinence seen.

Stage 7 a-f – Severe or Late Stage Dementia: Mostly **bedbound and incontinent.** Worsening ability to swallow and loss of speech. Unable to even sit, hold head up or smile in the last stages. Most patients in stage 7 will be hospice appropriate. Most die of complications of sepsis or pneumonia.

(Reisberg, 1998)

I then advise that patients may wish to choose any of the above levels as their minimum acceptable function and add it to their advance directives, in their own words. For example:

If I were to get dementia, then I do not want my life prolonged by any medicines or machines if:
I cannot recognize family members
Or if I have stopped talking and smiling
Or if I am unable to swallow and enjoy food, do not put me on feeding tubes
Or if I am totally bedridden and incontinent
And so on…

I warn the patients again about the non-beneficial aspects of feeding tubes as mentioned before.

I also urge people to think about, in the event of dementia, at what stage they may wish to be a DNAR, keeping in mind that if resuscitated after an arrest, they would be functioning at an even lower level than where they were before resuscitation. I explain that discussions with their physician are paramount to understand the pros and cons.

Here is sample wording from the end of life living plan of ADM, who is a 70-year-old grandmother who has had Parkinson's for four years but is managing very well and is totally independent:

If I should develop Alzheimer's or other Dementia and cannot recognize my loved ones or take care of myself or feed myself, I want ALL medications to be discontinued. Do not feed or hydrate me then but keep me quiet and comfortable until I fall asleep and die.

If I don't request food or water, do not feed me or hydrate me by hand.

Continue any treatments necessary for my comfort so I do not suffer.

I want to die quietly with family at home.

Reference:

Reisberg, B. Functional Assessment Staging (FAST*). Psycho pharmacology Bulletin.* 1988:24:653-659)

Goals of care

Drive

The plan of care

16 | MAKING DIFFICULT CHOICES: WHOSE RESPONSIBILITY IS IT? – DECISION VS RECOMMENDATION VS RECOMMENDED DECISION

I believe that physicians need to take a more proactive role in difficult decisions. To treat or not to treat and how to treat is first a medical decision.

At the beginning, the process demands that the physician contemplate the decision in light of the patient's best interest, based on best medical judgment, taking into account all the different medical and ethical factors and the pros and cons, along with the patient's culture, beliefs, goals, wishes and views.

This is then presented to the patient/family as a medical decision, all the while explaining the reasons why the decision makes sense and what good it would bring, looking for their understanding and agreement. If agreement is reached, great. If agreement is not attained, it is the physician's responsibility to further facilitate the family's understanding of the facts, answer further questions so that decisions are made with full information, including a **clear prognosis and progress with focus on goals**, the likely response to therapies and the most likely outcome. This is necessary to avoid misunderstandings.

If a joint decision with the patient/family is still not reached, consultation with a palliative care team or the ethics committee may be warranted.

This is the ideal scenario. Unfortunately, oftentimes the "hard" decisions are left totally up to the family, with very little guidance.

Here's the process in short:

- Contemplate what would be a good decision.
- Recommend it to the patient/family and explain why it is a reasonable decision.
- Look for understanding and agreement from the patient and family.
- Be open to other views, ideas, and reasons.

When someone comes to us with shortness of breath, we do not ask the patient to choose what studies he/she should have, or what antibiotics to give. But when there is a serious decision to make, like DNAR or withholding or stopping treatments, we tend to leave it totally in the hands of the family.

I have had physicians tell me that they will do whatever the family wants no matter what. Our job, however is to help in the decision-making process, using our experience and knowledge to light the way for them at this difficult juncture. Being the experts in the field, it falls upon us to be making the hard decisions, presenting them to patients and families, clearly giving reasons why those decisions would be the right choice for "this patient at this time given these facts."

While guiding families through this, you may say "our **recommended decision**" instead of just "recommendation" to emphasize what *we* think is medically appropriate. You may also say that "**medically and ethically**" this would be the right action. Again, give the reasons why. I usually say something like:

*Here is our **recommended decision**, here are the reasons why it makes sense and would be best for the patient, and also how the results are in keeping with what is important to the patient/family and the goals to be achieved.*

For example:

Your father has an end stage disease. He has lost his ability to make decisions and he is now totally dependent on others for all his daily needs. Since he has multiple organ failure (lungs, heart, and kidneys), his chances of surviving and going home after a cardiac arrest are almost zero. Even if we got his heart going, I am sorry to say he will not leave the hospital. He will be on life support until he arrests again, and again.

*It would be against all ethical and medical principles to try and resuscitate such patients since we cannot make them better. It will actually be causing more pain and suffering. Our **recommended decision** here is not to resuscitate in case his heart stops. We would therefore write a "DNAR" order for him; in other words, "do not attempt resuscitation in case of an arrest."*

*All treatments would continue unless your father has a cardio-pulmonary arrest. His care will never stop. I hope you understand and see the reasoning for **the recommended decision**. Our job is to help improve the life of our patients* *and decrease pain and suffering, not make it worse. I wish things were different, but I have to give you the facts as they are."*

When you are **recommending a decision,** and looking for agreement from the family/patient, it is more of an "assent" than a "decision" to make and is much less burdensome for both family and patient.

Most of the time, families know what the right decision may be, but are unable to say so because of the emotional burden it places on them. In an ethics committee consultation, a patient's nephew put it clearly on the physician's shoulders when he said, *"You guys are the experts, why don't you make a decision and tell us what to do?"*

Shared decision-making is ideally an all-inclusive concept. It works well if everyone is on the same page and have similar understanding, reasoning ability, and emotional connection. Even then, there can be a lot of differences of opinion based on multiple issues.

One would like to respect the patient or family's wishes and preferences as much as possible, but that in of itself cannot be the only driver of decisions. The decisions have to be rational, reasonable, and **of benefit to the patient.** It is not unusual for families to exhibit emotional irrationality at these times, especially if their decisions have to do with letting go, or foregoing life-sustaining treatments. The family members who have not been close physically or emotionally (the daughter from far away) seem to have even a harder time of letting go.

Do all available treatments have to be offered to all patients at all times?

The obvious answer is "no!"

Not all possible treatments have to be offered to every patient in all cases as a possible choice. Those that are clearly of no benefit can be mentioned but not recommended as a choice and can be taken off the table because they wouldn't achieve the desired goals.

For example, if you were talking to the daughter of a 75-year-old lady with end stage dementia you would say:

Your mother has end stage dementia and is now having difficulty swallowing. You are probably wondering about a feeding tube. Feeding tubes are not recommended at this stage in dementia since they do not improve health, prolong life, or decrease chance of aspiration. In addition, they can add more complications. Since they are of no benefit and may actually increase harm, they are off the table for consideration. Let's talk about what can be done to improve her comfort and quality of life.

Autonomy is important, but it can be overemphasized and demand too much of the patient or surrogate. Sometimes asking families to "make" major decisions at the end of life is unfair and very problematic. It is nearly impossible for some to make such decisions; for example, a loving spouse or a close family member who is emotionally connected to the sick and dying person.

Like the minister father said of his 40-year-old daughter with AIDS who was on life support: "I would not want to live like this, but she is my daughter. How can I agree to stopping life support and let her die? She is my daughter, man!"

Even giving all the information and just making a recommendation may not be enough.

Clinical situations in which withholding treatments is clearly warranted ought to be presented as medical decisions, rather than asking patient or family to make a decision. A clear example would be a DNAR for patients with multiple organ failure. Most patients and families tend to agree easily when presented with the facts.

Similarly, for terminal patients who continue to show deterioration in spite of aggressive therapies, physicians can, at the opportune time, decide not to escalate treatments or even to stop certain treatments if they are not contributing to achieving the agreed upon rational goals. This may include blood transfusions, dialysis, TPN, etc. The same is true for lab and radiologic studies. If they are not contributing to the improvement of the clinical status and helping achieve goals, then they can also be stopped.

In these cases, the patient/family needs to be informed with compassion and given proper explanations, and their questions and concerns must be addressed.

If the patient/family are not accepting, they have to be informed of their choice to find a different provider if they wish. Of course, they are at liberty to get a court order for providing certain treatments the physicians feel are futile. As I explain these options, I say something like:

If they were to obtain a court order, then we will provide those treatments even though we may think that they are medically and ethically wrong.

In over 25 years, our palliative care team has never had a family go to court for this. We have, however, had many of them thank us many times for making the decision so they did not have to.

The only caveat, in the state of Maryland at least, is that we cannot stop a treatment against a patient's/family's wishes that is going to result in immediate death of the patient. But there is a process to jointly achieve that. Two physicians may document that treatments are futile/inappropriate and give families a reasonable amount of time to find alternate providers before stopping life-prolonging treatments. In our institution, ethics committee consultation is also required in such cases for withdrawal of life support. Hospital administration's support is paramount. At our hospital the letter informing the family of the proposed action is signed by the VPMA or the CEO. The physician is not liable if he/she follows the ethics committee recommendations.

It is important to know the law in your own state. Your hospital lawyer or ethics committee chair can be a good source of information. In Texas, for example, physicians can stop life-sustaining treatments after they have agreement from the ethics committee and the family has been given ten days to find alternative care.

Medical DNAR

Physicians are under no obligation to provide treatments that are medically ineffective, non-beneficial, or ethically wrong. We need to help families understand the reasons why some treatments cannot be offered. It is our obligation to do what is right and "good" for the patient, and address the goals and limits of "shared decision-making" – the science and art that respects patient's values and preferences but recognizes limits due to emotional burden and cognitive challenges during illness.

Given a patient whose clinical condition indicates resuscitation will be of no benefit, physicians can decide not to resuscitate if a patient has a cardio-pulmonary arrest. Legally, in Maryland, two physicians, one being the attending on the case, can write justification for it and write a DNAR order as a purely medical decision. (Check your state and local laws and your hospital's policies). Family is informed of the decision and given reasons why this is the right action for the patient. Not resuscitating after a patient dies is a valid medical choice in treating a symptom or event when the physician has determined that the patient's overall health cannot be improved or the disease cannot be stopped.

Our actions are not resulting in the death of the patient. Rather, the patient is dying of natural causes and we are electing not to resuscitate, since now it is of no use given the patient's condition. And, of course, the patient and/or family is informed of the decision.

Yes, it takes some courage and confidence, but knowing that it is the right thing to do for the patient, we have to pursue it. It is our job and responsibility. Just as we would offer only useful treatments in treating cancer, we ought to offer only useful treatments at the end of life – the treatments that help achieve the rational and reasonable goals of the patient. If the patient/family disagree, they always have a choice to find new providers who are willing to resuscitate under these circumstances. In my experience, that rarely happens.

The following case illustrates how a medical DNAR can actually be a gift to the patient and family:

> J Jones was a 74-year-old gentleman with chronic heart failure. Two years earlier, he'd had a stroke, but had recovered to a functional level.
>
> Two months prior to this admission, he had pneumonia and sepsis which required intubation and vent support. He was unable to be weaned off the vent, so he ended up in the chronic vent unit at our hospital.
>
> Then, another bout of sepsis with UTI landed him in the ICU. He recovered enough to be sent back to the chronic vent unit, where a week later he arrested, was resuscitated, and then sent back to the ICU.
>
> Now, he was unconscious, showing signs of renal failure and on life support with vasopressors to keep him going. His wife continued to want him to be resuscitated again in case of an arrest, so a palliative care consult was called.
>
> I met with the wife and daughter and explained why resuscitation was now medically and ethically not indicated, and that the DNAR was a clear medical decision, saying:

"He has been resuscitated once already and continues to be resuscitated presently with the help of vasopressors, oxygen, and the vent. If, in spite of all of that, he arrests again – essentially dies – then resuscitating again does not make sense because it will not work.

Patients like these with such severe problems will never leave the hospital, even if we can get the heart going. They will arrest again and again until they die. This now is a medical decision and we cannot offer treatments that are of no use to a patient, and actually may cause more harm and suffering. Thus, we are going to make him a DNAR and if he dies we are going to let him go in peace."

The wife very calmly said she understood but did not agree and still wanted him resuscitated. The daughter was visibly distressed and crying quietly.

I said, "I am sorry, we cannot do what is of no use and may actually cause more harm. This will be ethically and medically wrong. We became doctors to help alleviate suffering, not cause more suffering.

Now you do have options if you want your husband to be resuscitated. You may transfer him to another hospital where they are willing to do this. As you know, you may get a court order that would compel us to resuscitate. In that case, we will comply even though we know it to be medically ineffective and ethically wrong."

After the meeting, I consoled the daughter since she was upset and the mother showed no signs of trying to comfort her. I again told the daughter that this was a medical decision at this point and they did not have to make a decision themselves.

She thanked me, hugged me, and said that she was glad we were making the decision so she would not feel guilty.

The patient had an arrest the next day and died. No resuscitation was done since we had made him a DNAR. If this had not been done, he would have had to go through this cycle again and again.

I see physicians too many times acquiescing to "whatever the family wants" even when it is clearly not the best course of action for the patient. This does take a little courage, but we need to stand up for what is our duty and is right for the patient.

The mere availability of a treatment or a procedure does not obligate you to offer it as an option

17 | HELPING SURROGATES MAKE DECISIONS

Once the patient has lost the capacity to make his or her own decisions, it falls to the POA for healthcare to make decisions. If there is no designated POA, then it falls to the surrogates in order of priority: a guardian, a spouse, an adult child, a parent, a sibling, a relative, and, then, a close friend.

Making EOL decisions for yourself is hard enough, but when you have to decide for your loved ones, the burden is just enormous. This is one of the hardest tasks a person faces.

Our job as physicians, again, is to help guide others, building a bond and a trusting relationship as we go. It is much harder with surrogates, and a tall order – but, if done with care and understanding, quite doable.

The following five "standards" can be helpful:
1. The Substituted Standard
2. The Best Interest Standard
3. The Reasonable Person Standard
4. The Gold Standard
5. The Commonsense Standard – The Quality of Life Issue

I'll explain each of these standards separately, sharing a few illustrative stories.

The Substituted Standard

When a patient's wishes are known, the surrogate is a simply a stand-in substitute, who will follow the wishes of the patient in all decision-making.

In order to use this standard, there must be a living will or an advance directive of some sort, or at least a discussion on EOL living goals between the patient and the physician, family, and/or surrogate. Most of the time, when I ask, the answer is, "no, we never talked about it."

It is important to talk to as many family members as possible to find out the patient's wishes, which is always helpful and at times crucial. I usually give the family "homework" – to go and ask as many friends and relatives as possible to see if the patient made any comments to anyone about EOL, because this may help us in deciding.

Yet again, we can see that having discussions with the family around "The Three Questions" is a gift the family leaves behind for the loved ones.

Story # 1: Jack and "Homework" for the Family

Jack was 78 years old and very weak and sick with heart failure. He spent most of his time just sitting in the chair and watching TV. Then he was admitted with worsening heart failure, sepsis, and kidney failure. He spent six days in the ICU on the respirator. Prognosis was very poor.

His wife wanted to continue with aggressive treatments, but the doctors felt it was time for more of a "comfort" approach.

Jack's wife was not aware of any of his wishes. She was given "homework" to do – to go home and ask ALL family members if Jack had ever made any comments regarding how he may have wanted to live –or not live – near end of life, which might guide us in deciding the course of action.

When we met the next day, her two sons accompanied her. They attested to the fact that their dad never wanted to be hooked to machines if he was not going to improve.

Since we were following Jack's wishes, the ineffective life-prolonging treatments were stopped without guilt on anyone's part, and he died with peace and dignity.

The family was also at peace that they were following his wishes, which came to be known even more deeply once most of the family was quizzed.

Story # 2: "I Do Not Want to Lie in a Bed of Affliction"

This is a true story which illustrates the fact that **just a simple comment in conversation can be helpful with difficult decisions later in life, even when there is no written advance directive or a living will.**

Mary was 93 years old, with mild dementia. She could let you know how she was feeling but could not make much sense otherwise, and could not make her own decisions. She had mild contractures of her legs and lay in bed most of the time, but could get up with help.

Mary was admitted with a painful left foot, gangrene of her toes, and sepsis. She was being treated with antibiotics. Doctors recommended amputation of the left leg below the knee to get rid of the gangrene.

Her family was asked for a consent, and her family members then met with the palliative care team to discuss options and see what would be the right choice. There were no written advance directives.

In further talking with Mary's family about the kind of life they thought she would have wanted to live, one of the sons remembered her saying, "I never want to lie in a bed of affliction."

The family was asked to keep this comment of hers in mind going forward and make decisions that would honor her wish of not lying in a bed of affliction.

With the help of this comment and the guidance of the palliative care team, they were able to decide not to have the surgery, because although that would give her a longer life, she would definitely be "lying in a bed of affliction."

They opted to enroll her in hospice instead and take her home to be with the family for as long as God wished her to be here. The family was at peace with their decision since they felt it followed Mary's voiced wishes.

Please encourage your patients to start having these talks about living and dying; what kind of life is acceptable to them and what is not. Even a casual remark about their preferences can be wind up being very helpful. **The key factor, and the beauty, is in having the talks.**

The Best Interest, Reasonable Person, Gold, and Commonsense Standards

When a patient's wishes are not known, the surrogate must use another standard to make decisions on behalf of the patient.

The Best Interest Standard refers to **doing what is in the best interest of the patient,** looking at all the burdens and benefits of the proposed treatments and management strategies, taking into account longevity and pain and suffering, as well as religious and cultural parameters that the patient would have followed as he/she made these decisions.

The Reasonable Person Standard invites the surrogate to ask **what a reasonable person would want** to do in this circumstance, a matter of discussion and debate.

The Gold Standard is to apply the golden rule; **treat others like you would want to be treated yourself.** Ask the family members to put themselves in place of the patient. I often ask surrogates something like:

"If it were you in place of your father, what would you do? In this situation, how would you want to be treated and why, given all the facts you know?"

This can be very helpful in making the choices more real for the decision-maker.

The Commonsense Standard goes straight to the **quality of life issue.** The important step for us is to **raise the question**. I just ask something like:

What do you think is the quality of life for your father now? Is he suffering? How would you describe it?

If the answer is poor or worse (I had a daughter say clearly about her father, *"Life? What life, he has no life!"*) and there is no chance of improvement, then one can concentrate on comfort and decreasing suffering.

DNAR would make sense since the patient will be in a worse state after CPR, and the suffering would be even greater. Stopping artificially life-sustaining treatments would also be appropriate, depending on the facts of the given case.

Another question I ask which I find helpful is this:

If your loved one were to go to sleep and never wake up, in other words, die, would you be ok with that? Will you be at peace?

If the answer is yes, then DNAR, and even stopping artificial life-prolonging treatments, may be appropriate. This means that the patient's present existence is so poor that allowing natural death would be preferable.

Many times, the family is unable to make a decision right then and has to be given time to think and talk to others who may not be there. Patience and gentle caring will go a long way in helping all.

Story # 3: At Peace

Alice, at age 87, was slowly becoming feeble. Now, after two years of decline, she could not talk, only grunt, and barely recognized anyone or smiled. She had also lost her ability to eat normally.

Her family was suffering, watching her in this poor existence. **Her three children all voiced that they would be at peace if she were to go to sleep and not wake up.**

The few cardiac meds that Alice was on were stopped, and she was offered food but not forced to eat. Comfort medicines were continued. She died a week later in peace with dignity. Her family was also at peace, knowing they did the right thing.

EMPATHIZE

EMPATHIZE

Empathize

Empathize

18 | LISTENING AND EMPATHY – THE GLUE THAT BINDS US!

Two of the top behaviors that help build a feeling of connection with patients and families are the art of listening and the skill of empathizing.

Although we have talked about listening and empathizing earlier, they are so important in relationship building, I'm exploring them a little further here.

Listening

Start with an open-ended request or question like "Tell me about your mother's life" or "How do you think your mother is doing?"

Then just listen, a lot more than you talk.

All patients have a story. Understand their narrative, and put them into context. Listen to their pain, hopes, and wishes.

Give them as much time as they need, without interruptions, so you may learn about them, their life, and what is important to them.

Physicians tend to interrupt patients about every 18 seconds! We need to learn to be great listeners, whether it is passive listening or active listening. (See the chapter on "Communication – The Key to Good Palliative Care, Resolving Conflict and Misunderstanding.)

When done well and combined with empathy, listening will bridge the gap, and you will start to build a relationship with this patient and family.

Here is an example of how to begin a "listening" conversation. Remember, after you say something like this, your job is to listen, both actively and passively:

"Before we can make any decision, and before I can help guide you towards the right decision which is "good" for your husband, I need to get to know him better. So, tell me about him first and then about his illness and the progress so far."

Empathizing

Empathizing is recognizing and affirming the emotion that patients or loved ones are exhibiting. You are, in the process, validating the emotion. And then you need to intellectualize it, which is to give reasons why they may be feeling this way. This lets them know that you see their emotion/distress and you understand the reasons for it.

This brings you closer to them, since the patient sees that you can notice their distress AND you understand why. This will also help build trust through gaining understanding.

Here are some examples of how empathizing sounds in action:

"I see that you are dismayed and disappointed to hear the results. That is totally understandable. You were not really expecting this. It looked like your dad may have been getting a little better, but he really is not. I'm sorry I don't have better news. His blood pressure has improved with the medications,

but the overall prognosis remains very poor because we cannot fix the underlying disease which has not responded to the treatments."

"You look so distressed. You have been married for 62 years. That is a long time. I see how hard it is for you to imagine a life without your dear husband after such a long time together. What is most important to you in the remaining time you have together? We are here to support both of you."

"I can see you are very angry and disheartened. I can see why. No one wants to lose one's parent. Even though we know we all must die one day, losing such an important person in our life is very hard. I wish I could make it all better, but unfortunately with so many complications the prognosis is not good. I am so sorry for your pain."

Take your time

Be tactful

Be honest

Be kind

Be gentle and caring

19 | BUILDING TRUST

Building trust is a very close second to listening and empathizing in building relationships, and actually happens as a result.

It is very simple. All you do is *keep your word.* How truthful and dependable you are in anything you say or do will help your patient's trust go up or down accordingly.

Even in simple little actions it becomes important. If you say you will come see the patient or meet the family at 3 pm, then, by George, be there by 3 pm. If you are running late even by 5 or 10 minutes, call to inform them. This little action will raise the trust even more. If you show up late by 10 minutes and do not inform them, the trust will go down, even if it is just a bit. So, keep your promises, be honest, be impeccable with your word and, do what you say.

DISAGREEMENT IS FROM MISPERCEPTION

CLOSE THE INFORMATION GAP

20 | MANAGING CROSS-CULTURAL ISSUES

As healthcare providers, we need to be aware that different cultures have different value systems. What is important to us may not be as important to others. People who espouse a different cultural worldview from ours are worthy of compassionate and dignified care as well. We need to know what that looks like across cultures.

It is impossible to know all the facts about all the world's cultures. Even the members of a culture may not agree on a given issue like autonomy or decision-making. Thus, the best approach to managing cross-cultural issues may be the following:

1. Be careful of your assumptions. You may start with broad assumptions, but be willing to let them go as you get to know this particular patient and family. It is good to know some basic information about different cultures but do not assume that the patient subscribes to it totally. Get the facts from the patient and family. Ask them, *"Is there anything I should know about your culture, religion, family, and values that may have a bearing on this? Please let me know. Don't hesitate to educate me. We want to do what is right for you and your personal beliefs."*

You may consider using Kleinman's eight questions for cultural assessment:
1) What do you think caused this problem/illness? What name does it have?
2) When and why did it start?
3) What do you think the illness does? How does it work?
4) How severe is it? Will it have a long or short course?
5) What kind of treatment do you think the patient should receive?
6) What are the most important results you hope the patient receives from the treatment?
7) What are the chief problems the illness has caused?
8) What do you fear most about the illness/problem?

2. Many Eastern cultures, like those from India, Pakistan, and the Middle East, may give more importance to beneficence and non-maleficence rather than autonomy. Decision-making may be deferred to others, many times to the eldest male of the family, whom they believe has their best interest at heart. Many females from those cultures may only want a female physician. Since we in America feel autonomy is so very important and a patient has a right to know and decide for himself/herself, we can just ask the patient whether they want to know the information/facts

themselves or do they wish for us to talk to someone else from the family and have them relate information and make decisions. This way we have given the right to make decisions to the patient, who has chosen how he/she wants the information and decision-making process to go. Thus, autonomy is safeguarded.

Case Study

Mr. KJ is a Muslim from India in the terminal stages of severe anoxic encephalopathy and heart failure. He does not have capacity to make decisions. His wife has the capacity to make decisions and legally is the surrogate decision-maker, but clearly indicates that she wants her son to make all decisions for her husband. She also cites examples where she and her son disagreed in the past, but followed the son's wishes. Although we always involved the wife in discussions, no decisions were final without the son's ok.

3. Oriental cultures tend to emphasize the emotional distress that bad news brings to a patient, and they may keep the patient a little in the dark from knowing a "bad" diagnosis, like cancer, so that at least emotionally they would suffer less and perhaps have a better, less stressful end of life. Thus, there is reluctance to discuss terminal diagnoses with the sick patient and we tend to

avoid terms such as cancer, terminal illness, and death. The belief is that the patient will be harmed by these discussions because he/she will be now in a depressed and in an anxious state. Not knowing the facts may actually give them a relatively better quality of life. (Ignorance is bliss.) If there is no foreseeable harm to the patient, the family's wishes can be easily followed.

Case Study

Maxine was a 56-year-old lady with metastatic colon cancer that had progressed to liver failure. The question of the futility of CPR was brought up to the family, but since Mary had capacity to make her decisions, she was approached with the question and given reasons why not resuscitating in case of an arrest made rational sense. She wanted to think about it.

When seen next day, it was obvious that she was having a very hard time deciding and would really rather not even think about it. She was asked if it would be ok to just talk to her family instead of her and let them decide. She readily agreed.

This took the burden off the patient, who was terminally ill to begin with and in much distress.

The family was given reasons why not resuscitating was the right choice and told that it was the medical team's recommended decision:

when there is no benefit to the patient, CPR is not done. The family could see the reasoning and readily agreed. This took the burden off the family's shoulders too. The patient's autonomy was respected and the family's burden lessened by being given a recommended medical decision and having the reasons explained to them.

4. Avoid cultural generalizations. Recognize the core issues listed below and explore them further with the patient, considering his/her own beliefs and preferences. These major areas in end of life treatment that vary socio-culturally are:

    a. Communication of bad news.
    b. The decision-making authority – for example, it is not unusual to find that the majority of Korean-Americans or Mexican-Americans are family-centered, while the majority of African-Americans or European-Americans are more autonomy-based in their decision-making.
    c. Attitudes towards advance directives, end of life care and aggressive life-prolonging treatments.

    d. The meaning of pain and suffering.

Many adults may feel that suffering is redemption and thus refuse to medicate themselves effectively against pain.

Case Study

A surprising case of this was a very caring father who was having difficulty appropriately giving pain meds to his four-year-old with terminal cancer because of his own strong belief that suffering was important for redemption.

After a very long discourse over hours, he did agree with the fact that probably there was not much that a four-year-old needed redemption for, so that giving medicine to decrease his child's suffering was not going to make him look bad in God's eyes. The child received better pain control after that.

Keep the focus on reasoning and on clarifying misconceptions. Making an effort to persuade someone to do the right thing is the way to go. You will need time and patience.

Be careful that your words do not come across as coercion, but more of a rational persuasion.

The father himself finally saw the light and said, "Yes, I see that at four years of

age he does not need redemption and we cannot let him suffer for the sake of others." He was then better able to provide pain control to his child.
    e. Gender issues. The roles of female and male might be clearly defined, and caution must be taken with regards to what is considered appropriate behavior.
5. Some of the reasons why families may wish not to disclose "bad news" to the patient include:
    a. It is considered disrespectful and impolite.
    b. Could cause more depression and anxiety which is an unnecessary burden and is negative emotionally.
    c. It will eliminate hope, then the patient cannot enjoy life anymore.
    d. It will make illness and death real, so it will have to be dealt with.
    e. It is cruel and inhumane to add this burden and additional suffering to the terminal patient.
    f. Acknowledging mortality may be self-fulfilling

Be careful when questioning patients about their beliefs and cultures so as not to embarrass, ridicule, demean or criticize their beliefs. Strive to use non-judgmental and sensitive language, such as:

"Since I am not well versed with your religion and culture, I would like to know, if there are any considerations we need to be aware of in order to honor your religion and values.

21 | ADDRESSING DNR/DNAR

First, it is preferable to use the term DNAR – Do Not Attempt to Resuscitate – which denotes that at best it would have been just an attempt with no assurance. DNR – Do Not Resuscitate – sounds like you could have been able to resuscitate but choose not to.

Among the tough end of life decisions, I have found that the ones relating to the DNAR are relatively easier to work through than those regarding the withholding or withdrawing of other life-prolonging treatments.

DNAR, DNR, No CPR, and AND (Allow Natural Death) orders come into play if the patient has a cardiac or pulmonary arrest.

Until that happens, the treatments that the patient is receiving will continue. If the patient arrests, the question then is, "Do we do CPR and support the breathing or not?"

The purpose of CPR is prevention of sudden unexpected death. CPR is not indicated in certain situations, such as terminal irreversible illness where death is expected.

Since the overall survival to discharge rate of all inpatient CPR is very low, we need to carefully choose whether to resuscitate or not.

However, DNR/DNAR should never signal the abandonment of the patient. Patients and families must be reassured that any treatments will continue until the patient's heart stops. Only then will CPR not be done, for the reasons discussed.

Although what the public sees on TV of CPR is very promising, close to a 75% success rate, the reality is far from that. Heart Disease and Stroke statistics from the American Heart Association for 2016, reported in *Circulation* and published on-line, indicate that for out-of-hospital cardiac arrest, the survival to discharge rate is about 12%, while for in-hospital cardiac arrest, the rate is 24.8%. The prognosis worsens with age and co-morbidities.

The success rate for out of hospital cardiac arrest in children is under 18%, with a survival to discharge rate of only 7.8%.

A study from Iran showed that for inpatient cardiac arrest, the initial success rate was 15%, but that the rate for those discharged alive from the hospital was only 10.6%, with full recovery in only 2%. (Goodarzi, 2015)

After-trauma success rates were a little better, close to 31.7% (with a 14.7% good to moderate outcome) for those requiring CPR only in the preclinical phase. If CPR was done in ER only, the survival rate was 25.6% (with good to moderate outcome in 19.2%). For those requiring CPR in the preclinical phase and the ER, only 4.8% survived and only 2.8% had a good to moderate outcome. (Zwingmann, 2016)

Other studies have quoted the incidence of CPR at 2.73 per 1000 admissions rates, with only 4-16% being discharged from hospital if CPR was done in the field and 18% for in-hospital CPR. (Hagihera, 2012; Ehlenbach, 2009)

There are three major ethical rationales for deciding CPR is not advisable:
1. **The chance that CPR will be successful is poor and the agreed upon goals cannot be achieved.** Either the treatment is not going to work at all or it may restart the heart, but we will not achieve the goal we hoped for (such as recovery to baseline, discharge from hospital, etc.). This is usually the reason for not administering CPR in severely sick patients with multiple organ failures.
2. **The quality of life before the arrest is poor.** If the patient were to arrest in this situation, then resuscitating and forcing him/her to live such a poor existence with the help of artificially life-prolonging treatments does not make sense and would not be right.

    This is generally assessed by simply asking the patient or family to tell you how they see the patient's quality of life. I have gotten the answers such as "He has no life," "This is not the Dad I knew," "He did not want to live like this," "it sucks," and so on. Families usually readily understand this and agree.
3. **Even though the present quality of life is somewhat acceptable, the resulting quality of life after resuscitation would be at a level that would not be acceptable to the patient.** If no conversations ever took place with the patient, then decisions are made on basis of what is in the best

interest of **the patient** and what a reasonable person would want.

Medically speaking, the treatment for cardiopulmonary arrest is to do CPR; ethically speaking, however, not all arrests have to be treated by CPR, especially if the result is not in keeping with the mutually agreed upon goals and/or if this will only prolong the pain, the suffering, and the dying process with little or no benefit.

The other unfortunate part of providing non-beneficial treatments is that it also prolongs the pain and suffering for the family. Medical staff also suffers, and giving non-beneficial treatments to patients is one of the reasons they experience moral distress.

Follow these simple ethical rules in medical decisions:

- Any and all actions have to be for the good of the patient.
- Define the good.
- See that the good is in keeping with the patient's goals, wishes, or values.
- Consider making a medical decision when therapies, including CPR, are clearly not beneficial, and give reasons to patient/family as to why not providing such treatments would be right, then look for agreement from patient/family.

Here's an example of suggested dialogue:

"*Many hard decisions have to be considered. My job here is to help you with the different choices and give you reasons as to why one makes more sense over the other so that you will be at peace that the right things are being done for your loved one.*

When someone is so sick, with multiple issues, two major decisions confront us. The first has to do with resuscitation in case of a cardiac arrest, in other words CPR, and the second has to do with aggressive treatments – whether to continue them or not and for how long.

The first decision is the easier of the two. At this stage, it is a medical decision. Patients with this severe end stage illness with sepsis and multi-organ failure are not resuscitated in case of an arrest.

The reason is that they will either not respond, or, even if we can get the heart going, they will never leave the hospital because they will arrest again.

Of course, the whole process of CPR can also be very undignified and traumatic to the patient.

After all this, we are still not going to be able to achieve our goal of improving the disease or his health.

I hope you understand why it makes sense to let him go in peace if he dies, in spite of all the treatments he is getting, which by the way will continue for now as is.

We are not talking about decreasing or stopping any treatments, only not resuscitating in case of death because it would be of no use, AND it will cause unnecessary pain and suffering to the patient ...and you all.

Sometimes I also add, *"We are here to help decrease pain and suffering, so doing things that only worsen or cause more pain and suffering is not good or right and it goes against what our role is. We became doctors to help alleviate suffering, not increase it."*

If the patient is on life support already (vents, vasopressors, dialysis, etc.), I would point out that he is already being partially resuscitated, so if he "dies" in spite of that, re-resuscitation does not make sense.

"If he continues to decline, then we may have to consider stopping life-sustaining treatments. Let us meet daily and confer. If there are other family members who need to come to see the patient or meet with us, let us plan for that now."

DANGERS of CPR

- Multiple interventions without attention to modesty
- Harm to patient from local trauma to ribs, lungs, etc.
- False hope by temporary restoration of heartbeat
- False hope by offering non-beneficial treatments
- Blinds the provider and patient from seeing the potential of palliation
- Resuscitation into a very poor state of existence
- May be followed by the complication of pneumonia, CHF, GI bleed, seizure, stroke, or renal failure
- Moral distress in caregivers who may be forced to take part in activity that they feel is ethically wrong

- Dissatisfying for the healthcare team in their work, knowing that what they are doing is of no ultimate benefit to the patient

The ritual of non-beneficial CPR cancels out good end of life care. Instead of the patient dying peacefully with loving family around, he/she dies with people pounding on the chest, giving electric shocks in a flurry of hectic activity.

Withdrawing or Withholding Life-sustaining Treatments

As stated earlier, this is the harder question and the more difficult decision. The reasons one would withhold or withdraw life-sustaining treatments are very similar to those for not resuscitating. **Ethically speaking there is no difference between withholding or withdrawing, but, emotionally, withdrawing is generally much harder for everyone concerned, including families and healthcare workers.**

So, let us be very clear as to what we want to achieve by those treatments before starting them. It is also helpful to put a time limit on trials of therapies before embarking on them.

The reasons for not starting or for stopping life-sustaining treatments would be:

1. The treatment is not working; there is continued clinical worsening despite all means of support.
2. The burdens of treatment outweigh the benefits. The quality of life will be poor afterwards, not what the patient would have wanted. (One example

would be the side effects of chemotherapy in terminal patients with metastatic cancer.) The quality of life is already poor and is not how the patient wanted to live, supported by artificial means. In other words, the burdens of the disease outweigh the benefits of continued survival.

References:

1. A. Goodarzi et al. Study of Survival Rate After CPR in Hospitals of Kermanshah: *Glob J. Health*: 2015 Jan; 7(1)52-58
2. J. Zwingmann et al. Outcome and Predictors for Successful Resuscitation in the Emergency room of Adult Patients in Traumatic Cardio-respiratory Arrest: *Critical Care* 2016; 20:282
3. 1 - A. Hagihera et al. Prehospital Epinephrine Use and Survival Among Patients with Out of Hospital Cardiac Arrest. *JAMA* 2012;307(11) 1161-1168
4. W. Ehlenbach et al. Epidemiologic Study of In-hospital CPR in the Elderly; *NEJM* 361; 1, July 2 2009

22 | MAKING THE FUTILITY TALK WITH PATIENT AND FAMILY EASIER – THE FUTILITY GRAPH AS A VISUAL TOOL

Utilizing a visual aid such as the "futility graph" or the clinical progress graph can be helpful in explaining to families the clinical progress and prognosis when recommending withholding, not escalating, or stopping life-sustaining treatment. The patient's health status as a percentage of normal is plotted on the y axis and time is plotted on the x axis. Major interventions can be noted with arrows.

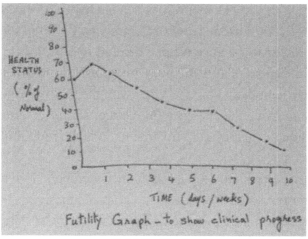

(Aziz) Futility Graph

I just hand-draw this on a piece of paper, as above, or on a whiteboard as I talk to the family. I tell them we are going to plot the **patient's clinical progress** on paper, so it is easily seen and understood.

I usually ask the family to tell me what % of normal health they think the patient had when he/she got admitted. They are always able to come up with a number, like 50%, 60%, etc.

Then I ask them to tell me where he/she was on succeeding days or weeks, as the case may be.

As they call out the percentages, I keep drawing on the paper or the board. I also add the major treatments as they occur in time to show how aggressively the patient is being managed.

As you can see, the graph above clearly shows that, despite aggressive therapies, the patient continues to worsen, and, thus, all we are doing is delaying the inevitable.

Seeing this in black and white can help drive home the futility of continued aggressive treatments. **Families can now see on the graph where we are headed to and thus grasp the poor progress and the poor prognosis more clearly.** This may help them come to grips with the reality, which can make some tough decisions a little easier and offer assurance that although we may stop treatments, it is the right thing to do.

If I am talking to only a few family members, I give them the paper on which I've drawn the graph so they can share it with the rest of the family to help explain the poor status.

Case Study

Herbert was an 83-year-old gentleman who loved nature and was a horticulturist. He loved being outdoors and worked in gardens with flowers and trees. He helped tend the National Arboretum and the White House gardens for a while as well.

Now, he had been sick for many months and presented to our hospital with septic shock, fungemia, respiratory failure, stroke, renal failure, and metabolic encephalopathy. He ended up on a respirator, vasopressors, and a feeding tube.

His wife died when she was young, and he just kept living with his in-laws. He took care of his mother-in-law when that became necessary and he never remarried. His decision-maker was Mary, his sister-in-law.

I talked with her and also his niece regarding the decisions that had to be made. They understood the multiorgan failure, the complications, and the poor prognosis.

I said, "You have a hard task ahead of you. Many major decisions have to be made. I am so sorry your brother-in-law has been so sick for so long. I am going to help you with these decisions, and give you reasons why possible treatments make sense or not.

"The first decision is the easier one, and that has to do with whether to resuscitate or not if Herbert's heart stops. Patients that have this much pathology, with multiple organs failing (lungs, brain, heart, and kidney) are not resuscitated if they have a cardiac arrest. The CPR will probably not work. And even if we do get the heart going, he will be in a worse state, and will never leave the hospital until he arrests again

and dies. We cannot give treatments that are going to cause more harm and suffering."

They readily agreed and understood the need for a DNAR order, as resuscitation would not be ethically and medically justified in someone with this much pathology and no chance of recovery.

I went on to say that the harder decision was the next one: What to do if he continues to show no improvement? How long to continue these treatments?

The sister-in-law voiced her dilemmas this way: "Should I let him go or not? How long should I leave him on the machine, since I know he did not want to live like this? Even sitting around was hard for him. He wanted to be up and about all the time. Am I playing God? Who am I to make that decision? I need to be unselfish."

I reassured her that we were not playing God. If it was not for us, he would have died by now. Are we playing God when we save lives? The disease was killing him, not our actions.

"Let's look at the course of his illness," I said, and drew the futility graph on paper with Mary picking the percentages for his health status, starting at 70% of normal, coming down gradually to 10% in 4 weeks' time.

"You can see where we are headed," I said. "This is despite us giving more and more of the aggressive treatments. His life is now maintained with the help of respirator, vasopressors, antibiotics, and G-tube feedings. We are only artificially sustaining life. If he did not want to live like this, then he essentially already made his decision. If we stop the artificial treatments and let nature take its course, then we will be honoring his wishes and it will be as God wanted.

Letting go is just as or maybe even more of an act of love and caring because you are doing it for him and not being selfish. A kind, loving, and dignified death is a gift for the one leaving us. It is part of life as we know it. Seeing the decline as I have shown you on paper in spite of very aggressive treatments tells us where we are headed. Not prolonging this unnecessarily with no hope of improvement would be the wiser, kinder thing to do. That would be our recommended decision. You are not alone in this. If this was a totally medical decision, we would have probably stopped the life support weeks ago."

Mary and her daughter seemed to agree but wanted to discuss it with the family.

We met again two days later. Her two uncles agreed, but Mary's mother had reservations, feeling we were euthanizing him like a dog.

I explained the difference between euthanasia (willfully administering medicine to end life) versus stopping treatments that were not beneficial and letting nature take its course, allowing natural death to occur.

I showed her the futility graph again to reassure her that our actions were unable to help make him better. Mary finally grasped the idea and was able to accept stopping non-beneficial treatments. Herbert died soon after he was taken off life support, finally at peace.

We were able to help Mary in her decision-making and she was finally at peace with it too, feeling very confident that she was doing the right thing. **Utilizing the futility graph to**

show the clinical progress helped her see with certainty what the future held.

23 | ADDITIONAL VISUAL TOOLS THAT ENHANCE CCOMMUNICATION

Seeing is believing. Make use of as many visual tools as possible, like pictures of **skin lesions, especially ulcers** (if the family has not seen the lesions on the patient or does not want to see them in person), lab data, **radiological data**, x-rays, CT scans, MRIs, etc. to show the severity and extent of the tumor/disease.

When trying to impress upon families the severity of skin ulcers, I ask if they have seen them. If not, I ask if they would like to see them to get a better idea. If not, I at least show them a picture or two so they understand what we are dealing with.

Our palliative care team also uses the **FAST Staging, the functional assessment for dementia's written hard copy**. It is shown to the family so they can judge for themselves as to the severity of the disease state.

It does have a big impact and they get a much better picture **seeing all this** instead of just hearing about it. As described above, I routinely draw the futility graph to show the decline and the proof that our continued efforts are in vain. I would highly recommend making use of any and all of these visual tools.

Mostly listen, and listen, and listen

Speak very little

and

then only with compassion,

clarity,

and consideration

24 | ENVELOPE DNAR/POCKET DNAR FOR CHILDREN

In pediatric hospice patients in the home, where parents may not be quite ready for a DNAR order on their child, our hospice and palliative care team has utilized what we call an Envelope or a Pocket DNAR.

Essentially, it is a DNAR order on the MOLST or POLST-like order form, signed by a physician and given to the parents to have and use if they so desire when the need arises.

The reason for this is that if the patient worsens and arrests, and parents decide that they now do not want CPR to be done, there will not be time enough to get an order to them. Then the child would get resuscitated and go through unnecessary suffering.

We instituted this Envelope or Pocket DNAR after having gone through a couple of such unfortunate events.

Most of the parents go along with it and feel secure that they have a choice. A few, who strongly opt for CPR no matter what, refuse to have one, although even if they did, they would not have to use it. If this form is not shown to the EMS personnel, CPR will be attempted.

GIVE

REALISTIC

HOPE

25 | THE HARD TALKS WITH PARENTS AND CHILDREN

These difficult conversations have to be done with parents and children too, when a child has a life-limiting illness. ***Our responsibility is not only the child, but the family.*** It is not unusual to see psychosomatic issues in the siblings who many times may feel sidelined since all the attention and time is given to the sick child.

Palliative care starts at the time of diagnosis of life-limiting illness, even prenatally in some cases. It can be provided right along with curative therapies.

Many patients enter palliative/hospice care too late. The "surprise" question may help – *Would you be surprised if your patient was to die in the next 6-12 months?*

If the answer is no, you would not be surprised, then a referral for palliative/hospice services is appropriate. If you are not sure, just have a phone consult with your local hospice or palliative care service.

Basic principles, the words we use, and how we approach the conversations stay the same as discussed elsewhere in this book. But for pediatric cases, the key point to remember is that children are not just small adults. Most of the talks happen with parents, but the manner in which children are involved depends upon their age and maturity.

Needless to say, it is a much harder dialogue, since a child's dying is out of the normal circle of life. You cannot imagine anything harder. And, yes, it is a mutual dialogue, not a one-way talk.

We cannot help others if we do not know where they are, how they think, and what they feel, hope, wish, or fear. The importance of asking, then listening and empathizing, is so very important in building bridges and bonds with the child and family.

Grief is immense. Emotions are high. Everyone is suffering. Everyone is trying to protect the other. So many times, communication among family members and with the sick child is not open, honest, and forthcoming. Conflict is not unusual.

If the basic relationships are not strong, the danger of families falling apart is very real. *Multi-disciplinary teams are a godsend in pediatric hospice and palliative care.* The work that the chaplains, social workers, nurses, bereavement councilors, and volunteers do in addition to the work done by clinicians cannot be underestimated. *Helping the child, siblings, and other family members deal with the unfortunate events takes a village and many approaches and modalities, like art, music, animal, and play therapy.*

Children need to be involved in the discussions and decisions depending upon their age and developmental stage. (Please refer to AAHPM's publication of Essentials Learning Module # 7)

Teenagers need to be given honest information and need to be involved in their choice of treatments (or not), setting goals to be achieved and for quality of life. I have found both the CPR/No CPR/DNAR decision, and the choice of treatments, including restrictions, much more rational and easier when the teenage patient was involved in discussion.

School-age children mostly want to be in school, play with friends, and experience new things. Every effort to help them achieve these goals needs to be made.

Very young children need family presence and closeness and touch for comfort and reassurance. They also need opportunities to express their feelings and ask questions. The team members from chaplaincy, social work, and child-life areas are priceless in this regard. Answers ought to be factual, in words they can understand, staying away from euphemisms, for example:

When one dies (not goes away), the heart and lungs stop working, and one does not suffer with pain or hunger. One does not come back. But one is at peace.

We have to keep reminding the parents that decisions are for the child, giving him/her as much of a positive experience as possible. Are the decisions good for the child? What is he/she getting out of this? How much positive, how much negative?

The sad cases are those in which the children have severe illnesses with neurologic damage or degeneration and have lost all ability to eat, interact, and in some cases even breathe, and are now being artificially fed by tubes and breathing with the help of a ventilator. The child is clearly not getting anything out of living like this, and suffering, but the parents cannot let go.

Some kids are at home on vents. This situation requires multiple, gentle, compassionate family meetings with all disciplines to help parents to let go for the child's sake, reassuring them that both choices – to continue or to forgo life-sustaining treatments – are loving choices.

"Let us see," we might say, "which one serves the child best at this stage."

All members of the team play a crucial role here in lending the necessary emotional support to help the family move forward.

We meet the parents where they are emotionally and work with them. The process of making major end of life decisions is slower, much more intensive, and more emotional on the part of the healthcare workers and, of course, the parents.

Parents need to feel that they were a good father/mother and did all they could for their child. In that zeal, sometimes we may see a child suffer unnecessarily with treatments which are not bringing him/her any benefit. **Concentrate on supporting parents in doing what can be done to make life a little more comfortable, peaceful, and less anxious for the patient.**

Helping parents feel fulfilled in their role with supportive, compassionate, and empathic responses becomes our responsibility. Helping parents and families through this time is a major part of our work. One might say, for example:

"You have been such a wonderful parent. What matters most to you now? What are you hoping for? What are your fears?"

Are we offering artificially life-prolonging treatments too readily in just about any kind of a case, even where life is not meaningful to the child? And are we under obligation to do so?

It is relatively easier to withhold futile treatments than to withdraw them. Patients with neurodegenerative diseases can survive for a long time if you support their breathing with a machine and nutrition by tube feeds. Since the heart is in good shape, they will probably die of an infection (pneumonia, sepsis, etc.) if not treated with antibiotics; but if you do, they would probably last a long time. The question for us is, did we serve the child well? If not, what are we to do in the future?

Some serious soul-searching and courageous conversations need to happen with clear, rational, achievable goals and honest laying out of the possible harms ***before*** we embark on these long-term, artificially life-prolonging treatments.

(Please refer also to Chapter 31, "Lessons Learned…" to hear the views of those working with children.)

COMMUNICATION IS THE HEART

OF PALLIATIVE CARE

26 | CUTTING TO THE CHASE – CLINICAL ETHICAL DECISION-MAKING: THE FASTEST WAY TO COME TO THE BEST DECISION FOR THE HIGHEST GOOD

Clinical ethical decision-making asks the question "why?" Why are we doing this test? Why are we giving this medicine or administering this treatment?

AND

    a) How is this treatment "good" for the patient? what is that good?

AND

    b) Is it in keeping with the patient's wishes, goals, values, and beliefs?

If the answer is yes all the way through, it is ethically the right decision.

Goals goals

GOALS

GOALS GOALS GOALS

Goals goals goals goals goals

GOALS GOALS GOALS GOALS

It's the goals that matter

27 | GOALS AND THE QUALITY OF LIFE

It is the goals that matter the most. Our conversations should be to first clarify those goals and the quality of life the patient wishes to get to, rather than get bogged down in the minutia of all kinds of treatments.

Once the goals of care are clear as to the type of life the patient wishes to live, then the plan of care (what treatments to give to get to the goals) becomes easier. If goals cannot be achieved, then withholding or withdrawing treatments becomes an easier and clearer decision as well.

Of course, some of the goals may be totally impossible given patient's condition. That is why the minimum acceptable levels of living (mental and physical, as discussed earlier in the chapter on "Advance Care Planning for End of Life in the Inpatient Setting – "The Three Questions...") become so important in defining the quality of life that is still good for the patient.

Examples of Goals from Some Patients

- I want to see my grandson graduate from college.
- I want to make it to my 90^{the} birthday.
- As long as I can recognize my family and verbally talk to them, any and all treatments are okay.

- Do not artificially prolong my life if I cannot communicate or I have severe dementia and do not know what I am saying or doing.
- I want my son not to suffer any more so please end his suffering and stop artificially prolonging his life.
- I do not want to lie in a bed of affliction.
- If I cannot swallow and enjoy my food, I do not want any artificial means of prolonging life.
- I do not want to live on machines.
- I have had a good life and no regrets. I am ready. I want to go if it is time to go, so I want to be a DNR/DNI.
- I want no treatments if I am not making sense mentally.
- If I am a quadriplegic and cannot make my decisions, I do not want my life prolonged by medicines or machines. Do keep me comfortable though.
- I would like to dance at my grandson's wedding before I die.
- I want to be a DNR if I have dementia and cannot have a meaningful conversation.

28 | FURTHER EXAMPLES OF END OF LIFE LIVING GOALS AND PLANS

All the following advance care planning examples were created by actual persons who are family members, friends, neighbors, and patients. The names have been changed for the sake of privacy.

As described earlier, most of the conversations revolved around The Three Questions to establish minimum levels of functioning that was acceptable to them if their life was to be prolonged by some artificial means in the future (medicines, machines, artificial nutrition/hydration).

This of course would only come into play if they became unable to make their own decisions and the family and physicians had to rely on their voiced/written preferences.

I hope you can see how simple and easily understandable these documents are. I advise those who have filled the state forms on advance directives to add these wishes and plans to their living will or advance directive documents, making that document even better. Otherwise, just create a new document for this information.

Names and minor details are changed to preserve confidentiality.

Example 1: ACP on a Well Visit

Sam was a 63-year-old Asian physician in fairly good health who wished to work on his advance directive. We worked on the three questions and his preferences are as follows:

1. I do not wish to be kept alive by means of any medicines, machines, or tube feedings **if I cannot smile, or I cannot recognize and communicate with my family or I cannot swallow, thus unable to enjoy food.**
   If I am in such a sorry state as described above, please stop all life-prolonging treatments (life-prolonging medicines included), but keep me comfortable and let me die in peace with dignity, preferably at home.
2. If the doctors feel I can be improved to whereby I can swallow, know my family, and communicate with them and smile, then I am willing to take aggressive treatments **only as long as I am showing positive improvement.**
3. Please always treat my pain and other symptoms so that I may not suffer.

Example 2: Preparing for Dementia

Joan is a 70-year-old Caucasian female with newly diagnosed Parkinson's disease. She can still function very well, and her symptoms are well controlled on medication. She is very worried about dementia and wants to control her living with it on her own terms. Her end of life living goals and plan is as such:

1. I have also filled in the "5 Wishes" and I want the specifics in that document to be followed along with this document.
2. I want to die quickly with the least indignities possible. I do not want to be seen and remembered in a sad, pitiful state.
3. If I should develop dementia and cannot recognize my loved ones or take care of myself or feed myself, I want all medications discontinued (except for those meant for my comfort).
4. I do not want to be fed or hydrated if I do not ask for it, but I want to be kept quiet and comfortable until I fall asleep and die quietly with family at home.
5. If I am paralyzed from the neck down, I do not want to be kept in that state even if I can communicate.
6. I do not want any life support if I have severe brain damage, in coma or close to death with an end stage or terminal condition and no hope of recovery.

7. I wish to donate all my organs and tissues.
8. I wish to be cremated and my ashes buried near where my family can visit as they wish.

Example 3: Oral Advance Directives

Mr. Golden is an 86-year-old gentleman with multiple comorbidities that include diabetes, coronary artery disease with heart failure, pneumonia, and kidney failure. Advance care planning was done in the presence of his two daughters and our palliative care nurse. The Three Questions to establish minimum acceptable levels were asked, as he had capacity so was able to make his own decisions. His wishes are as follows:

1. He does not want his life prolonged by any treatments if he is unable to recognize his family **and** communicate with them.
2. He also wishes no curative treatments if he is totally bed bound or unable to eat and swallow.
3. He is willing for short term intubation if it can help him achieve the level of function as described above in #1.
4. He does not want to be resuscitated if he has a cardiac arrest.
5. Dialysis and other treatments are ok only if it will help him achieve the mental awareness level as described in #1 above and keep him from being totally bed bound and dependent.

6. He wants only comfort care once it is clear that the minimum levels cannot be achieved (#1).
7. He wishes to die at home when that time comes.

In this case, I signed the progress note and our nurse signed as the witness, essentially agreeing that the discussion took place and the content is true. This is now an oral advance directive.

We made copies and gave them to the family.

Example 4: A Physician's Wish

Dr. Prakash was a physician of Indian decent. He had multiple cardiac, respiratory, and liver ailments. When seen by me for his advance care planning and goal-setting, he was in the ICU but had capacity to make his own decisions. I met with him at his own request to talk about end of life wishes and living plan. The summary of his wishes is as follows:

1. In case of a cardiac or respiratory arrest, there is to be no resuscitation. Let me go in peace.
2. If I, Dr. Prakash, lose my mental capacities so that I am unable to make my own decisions, I do not want my life extended by artificial means (such as medicines, machines, or artificially given food or water).
3. If I cannot perform activities of daily living, I do not want my life prolonged by artificial means either.

4. I want to be treated as long as there is a chance to get me to my goals as mentioned in #2 and #3 above.
5. If ever treatments are stopped, I want to be kept comfortable and die in peace with no suffering.

This document got signed by Dr. Prakash himself and two unrelated witnesses, a social worker and a medical resident.

This is now a legal document and copies were made and given to all concerned. It is interesting to note that a physician chose a very high mental function as his lowest tolerable level. Perhaps he has seen what may happen when others are deciding for you and does not want to leave anything to chance.

Of note also is that, in my conversations with other physicians compared to non-physicians, most tend to want a very high mental function as their lowest acceptable level for use of life-prolonging treatments.

Example 5: Goals of Care driving the Plan of Care

Lori was a 91-year-old lady with multiple ailments involving the heart, lungs, and kidneys, along with diabetes. She was recovering from a bout of pneumonia. The palliative care team was consulted to establish clear goals of therapy so that a plan for care could be formulated.

Lori had capacity; thus, the decisions were made by her, in front of her daughter, with our guidance. She was very clear about her goals of care, and they were as follows:

1. The ability to converse with her daughter.
2. Being able to enjoy food orally and not wanting any artificial feeds.
3. Comfort was prime.
4. Quality of life to be at least as described above.
5. She was at peace with herself and life, so if she was to go to sleep and never wake up, she was ready, as was her daughter.

PLAN OF CARE:

Once the goals were clearly defined, we were able to make the plans for her care. These were all agreeable to the patient and her family and were as follows:

1. Make the patient DNAR and DNI (do not intubate).
2. No artificial feeds (IV or tubes).
3. Try oral pleasure feeds as tolerated.
4. Hospice consultation.
5. Send home under home hospice with no return to hospital.
6. If gets infections, treat at home as necessary for comfort.
7. If loses capacity to converse, stop all life-prolonging treatments, but make sure she does not suffer.
8. Even if other treatments are stopped, comfort care will always continue till the end.
9. Offer family support as needed to help with grief and loss.

You can see how helpful it is to clarify goals first, because then the treatment choices can be made to adhere to the goals that are important to the patient.

Example 6: Autonomy – Listen to the Patient

A palliative care consult was requested of us to advise on the appropriate course of action on a patient who was refusing to take his medications.

Earl was a 67-year-old inmate from a nearby prison. He was in the end stages of terminal pancreatic cancer and in severe pain. Our conversation took place in the presence of two correctional officers and the social worker.

Earl put his story as such and I quote, *"No light at the end of tunnel. It's rough. Let me die. It's not how long you live, it's the quality of life. Quality of life is not good. I am in pain."*

("And so is your family," I added.)

"Let me go and let me die. It's not all about me. They act like I am crazy. I am not. I am not cursing staff or anything like that. I put myself here and I am peaceful. I want to take myself out. Nothing is wrong with me (mentally). I am just lying here in bed. I need pain medicine.

"There are a thousand miles, today is the first step."

The more we listened to Earl voice his hopes and wishes, the clearer the course of action became.

Earl cried, was dejected and in obvious emotional pain. It was clear that he was lucid, had capacity and was making rational decisions and requests.

After further discussions with Earl the following recommendations for the plan of care were made, keeping his wishes in mind:

1. DNAR and AND (no attempt at resuscitation and allow natural death).
2. Stop all tests and curative treatments.
3. Aggressive palliative therapy to be given and involve hospice services.
4. No artificial nutrition and hydration.
5. Discharge ASAP to be in a comfortable place in the institute (they had beds available).
6. Meet with family to explain plan.

All this was detailed in progress notes, signed by me, and witnessed by the nurse. This now is his oral advance directive.

Copies were given to patient and family and the MOLST [Medical Orders for Life-Sustaining Treatments] form filled out accordingly.

Earl's wishes were followed, and he was sent back to the institution under comfort care protocol.

Use your words
carefully.
   They are the best tools
you have
to soften the blow
  of the unkind reality
of the tragic winds of
fate.

29 | WORDS, WORDS, WORDS!

*"Words are both better and worse than thoughts; they express them and add to them; they give them power for good or evil: they start them on an endless flight, for **instruction**, and **comfort** and **blessing** or for **injury, sorrow,** and **ruin**."*

- Tyrone Edwards

It's what we say and how we say it that matters. Kind words uttered with understanding and compassion can go a long way in easing the pain of loss and helping others bear the burden of difficult decisions.

Words can hurt or heal. Use your language carefully. It is the best tool you have to soften the blow of the unkind reality of the tragic winds of fate.

1. **Avoid saying "There is nothing more we can do."**

    It signifies hopelessness and maybe even abandonment. It is an incomplete sentence by itself. Focus on the positive, what we can do rather than what we cannot do. There is always something we can do.

    Consider saying, *"There is nothing more we can do to cure the cancer, or to get rid of the disease now, but there is a lot we can do to help with the pain, breathing and to take care of you.*

We can focus on making the remaining time as good as possible and working on the achievable goals as you would wish now."

2. **Avoid saying "Do you want everything done?"**
Who would not want everything done? This question is vague and too broad. We need to be more specific, with focus on the goals.

Conversely, when a patient says, **"I want everything done," that is also an incomplete sentence**. Want everything done to achieve what? What are the goals to be achieved by doing "everything" and what does 'everything" entail?

Ask in response, *"So you want everything done. What does that mean to you? What is it that you are hoping to achieve? What goals do you wish to attain? Let us see if we can help you get there."*

If those goals cannot be achieved by doing "everything", then the proposed or requested treatments are futile, of no benefit since they will not help get to the desired goals and thus do not have to be offered.

A physician is under no obligation to provide treatments that are either medically ineffective or non-beneficial (cannot help achieve the desired mutually agreed upon rational and reasonable goals) or ethically inappropriate.

3. **Avoid saying *"It's time to pull the plug"* or *"it's time to pull back."***
   Consider instead, *"It's time to talk about the future management. Looks like we cannot reach the goals that we were hoping for."* (Give factual information).
   ***"Goals will shift** from trying to reach for a cure to concentrating more on comfort care and, with the help of a team of experts, managing pain and suffering as well as we can. **Any and all treatments that are beneficial will continue.** Those that are not helpful will be stopped. We will continue to help and care for you to improve your quality of life as best as we can."*

4. **Avoid saying "We are running out of options."**
   Consider, *"We are running out of options for cure. Let us talk about what is important to you now and see what further goals you want to achieve. What are your hopes and wishes for the future?"*

5. **Avoid saying "The patient is getting better."**
   Especially when this is not true for the overall picture. Avoid the word "better" by itself. Clarify. Keep the focus on the overall picture and prognosis.
   Consider saying instead, *"Although some parameters such as blood pressure and oxygen*

saturation show improvement, overall prognosis is still very poor given the multiple comorbidities and worsening of the cancer..."

When families hear the word "better" they feel it is all going to be well now. Then, when you start talking about DNR/DNAR/AND/NO CPR or withholding/withdrawing treatments, there is a disconnect and it is very hard for them to accept since they did not expect it.

If they continue to hear the poor prognosis and especially any deterioration in the clinical condition no matter how small, getting to acceptance is a little easier. They will be a little more prepared and it will be less of a shock or disappointment.

6. **Avoid saying "I know how you feel."**

It is impossible to know how someone else feels in a difficult stressful situation. The patient's response may be "How could you know how I feel? You're not the one with the cancer diagnosis."

But you may acknowledge their emotion and even reason out why they could be exhibiting that emotion.

Try saying something like, *"I see that you are frustrated and angry. This is understandable since every time you see an improvement, there is another complication and the condition continues to worsen overall. So frustrating. You have been dealing with this for a good 6 months and it is so hard to see your child suffer so..."*

This is empathizing. It lets them know that you see what they are feeling and why you think they are feeling that way. It's a strong communicating technique that builds bridges between the patient, the family, and you, the physician. It's a great skill to have. Practice it so you are comfortable and use it as often as possible.

7. **Avoid saying "You cannot give up hope."**

Consider instead, *"We can hope for the best but also prepare for the worst in case things do not go as planned."*

Give realistic hope. Explain problems at hand, the response to treatments, the progress of the patient and your reasons why the prognosis is as you describe.

Avoid giving false hope by offering treatments and procedures that are of no use. The mere availability of a procedure or treatment does not mean it has to be offered as an option to all, every time. By continuing to do more and more procedures/treatments, we may be giving an erroneous message.

As long as we keep doing more treatments and more procedures, we give the impression that some good is going to come of it. If we cannot get to the patient's desired level of existence, all these therapy options are unethical. The use of G-tube in end stage dementia is a good example of that. CPR in a patient with multiple organ failure is another.

Hope never ends but it changes in time. From hope for cure, it goes to hope for a long survival, to hoping for a few more months or till next birthday, or next Christmas, to few more weeks to days, to one more smile, to hope for a painless existence, to a pain-free death.

As the father of the 17-year old boy with brain tumor said as he lay in bed with his son, "I am just waiting, my hope is for the Lord to take him gently now."

Ask the patients and families what they hope for. But be as realistic as you can be. I often say that as we hope, let us keep praying. It always gives me comfort. See if you can help patients achieve some of what they hope for.

8. **Conversely, *don't* avoid mentioning death.**

Use the "D" word. If a patient is going to die, use the word death. It makes it more real. It's hard to process the concept if you don't hear the word. Be culturally aware, though, of what words may be a no-no in some circles.

I recently had to go home to Pakistan after my sister died. While there, I worked with many of the family members on their advance directives and end of life living plans for the future. While working with my brother on his documents that mentioned death, he got really quiet and, with trepidation, mentioned that he would prefer we did not use the word death but wrote something else like "passing on," etc. "Death seems so final," he said. "Passing on is more like going onto the next life..."

I often ask families to keep praying for whatever they wish for. Many times, I will pray with them to help find solace and peace.

9. **Avoid beating around the bush.**

    We try to soften the blow by not being totally honest and presenting a picture not as dismal as it really is. This does not work. Be kind, but be honest and truthful, and give the facts. It's hard to make good decisions with half the facts.

    If organs are failing, **use the word failure**: heart failure, kidney failure, lung failure, skin failure, brain failure, etc. Hearing the word failure has a more realistic effect than just "not functioning," "not up to par," or "below norm."

    More than once, I have had families who wanted to keep everything going until they heard that organs were "failing." They actually would remark," Oh, we did not know his organs were failing!" Then they were able to agree to a less aggressive approach and make more realistic decisions.

Every situation is different, including a host of different cultures, religions, and belief systems. Take time, be tactful, be honest and caring.

10. **Avoid using the "H" word.**

Apart from death, **hospice** is the other word patients and families do not like to hear. Instead, describe what hospice is in your own words like: *"How about if we now get a multidisciplinary team consisting of folks with varied backgrounds (doctor, nurse, social worker, chaplain, volunteer, bereavement counselor) to help you manage the rest of your illness at home? You would not have to run to the hospital for every problem and you would have a 24/7 on call nurse to call if necessary.*

They would come to your home and assist in helping take care of you and your family's needs. They would support all with psychosocial issues and help in alleviating physical, emotional, and spiritual issues." Most patients like the idea and wish to receive the help.

We agree, commenting, *"Yes, it is a wonderful service and it is called hospice. We will get their liaison person to come and meet with you for an informational meeting, to explain as to what they do and how this would work. You can decide to enter hospice or not after you have had all the pertinent information. We recommend it highly, but it is your decision.*

11. **Avoid talking about what you cannot do. Concentrate on what you can do.**

    "We can improve quality. We can decrease unnecessary suffering, we can help improve comfort. There is hope for decreasing pain along with emotional and spiritual suffering. We may not be able to extend life, but we can help make this remaining time as good as possible."

End of life experiences linger with the family; where and how these experiences happen are very precious for them

30 | LESSONS LEARNED – A ROUND-UP OF TIPS AND INSIGHTS FROM PHYSICIANS AND PALLIATIVE CARE TEAM MEMBERS

I questioned a number of my colleagues from many disciplines, including physicians, nurses, nurse practitioners, social workers, ethicists, chaplains, and bereavement counselors as to what important lessons they learned as they visited with their patients and families and what they consider to be high on their list of how to have these conversations on end of life issues.

Here are some of their responses:

Grace H – Hospice and Palliative Care Physician:
- It's about the patient and their goals, not your knowledge. Patient centered.
- Present in a positive way.
- Death is normal. If we can normalize this, we will all become much more comfortable having these talks.

Steve W – Hospice and Palliative Care Physician:
- Conscious plan not to talk but listen instead. Ready to ask questions and listen before talking. Don't be afraid to use the "D" word.
- I wish statements – tactfully done:
"I wish we could offer something else, I wish the oncologist had other good options etc."
These I messages are very helpful when you are being empathic.

Carlos Z – Director of Palliative Care:
- Educate patient and family first about the primary disease, the disease process and expected course. This is especially critical in dementia. It is the dementia resulting in complications of pneumonia and skin ulcers and not the other way around.
- Physicians, including specialists like oncologists, neurologists, cardiologists, and nephrologists, etc. need to clearly lay out the disease's path and give truthful evaluations as the condition worsens. Very often, and it happens a lot, the family never realizes how severe the problem is until they talk to the palliative care team. This makes me think that the previous docs are not giving the full picture factually. The specialists need to have more realistic talks earlier in the game. It would also make the role of the palliative care team easier.

Sarah B – Palliative Care Nurse Practitioner:
- The less I talk, the better the meeting.
- First talk about the disease state as patient/family understand it.
- Concentrate on the most important goal to the patient/family.
- Take burden away from the family by (physicians) making the hard decisions.
- Use a hard copy of a FAST staging sheet to help family see the severity of the dementia.

Chris K – Director of Palliative Care:

Communication is the heart of palliative care. The following words and actions I have found to be very helpful:
- Patient is the center of this, he is the boss, keep him in mind always.
- Providers need to get on the same page.
- We are working together with family and patient, making shared decisions.
- Be honest about realistic choices available.
- I say to families that they have a second responsibility to protect the loved ones from us (the medical industrial complex).
- There is a limit to how far we can go. We are human beings, taking care of another human being. We are not God.
- Silence is a powerful tool.
- Trust is not automatic but can be earned.

- Deepen the question to gain understanding when they say something by asking, "Tell me more."
- Use respect and be respectful. Ask, "Are you surprised by what I am saying? and "Do you think your loved one is suffering?"

Anita T – Clinical Medical Ethics Consultation and Research:
- When trial of therapies is given, clear goals and expectations need to be set in terms of time and stopping parameters.
- EOL decisions are not just about code status, but people's needs.
- In dying patients find the least bad way to die.
- Physicians need to take a leadership role in EOL decision-making.
- Involve legal counsel sparingly.
- Use ethics committees freely.

Caren G – Pediatric Hospice Pediatrician:
Help families reframe hope: hope to create new memories, hope for less pain, hope for gentle passing.

Heather S – Pediatric and Neonatal Hospice Social Worker:
- When conversing about DNR/DNAR discuss in a manner that gives parents control about making decisions.

- Bonding increases while talking of other things besides the illness, and being genuinely not in a hurry.
- My favorite question to parents is, *"Tell me about her when she was not sick – back to the good times."*
- Talk to siblings away from the parents.

Barbara A – Pediatric Hospice Social Worker:
- First priority is to make a connection with family.
- Most important goal in communication about goals of care is to meet the patients and families where they are!
- Ask for and listen to their perceptions of how their child is faring, what is most important to them, what they expect to happen, and what has been done so far.
- Timing of the various conversations is important.
- Ask permission to share your views.
- Give information in small bits so as not to overwhelm.
- It is an on-going process, moment by moment, what the family is ready to hear.
- Imperative to use skills of active listening, validation, empathy, and cultural humility.
- Be respectful of cultural and family needs.
- Help families in talking to children in a developmentally appropriate manner.

Geoff C – Hospice Medical Director:
Sit down, relax, act like you have all the time in the world. Turn off the cell phone.

Nancy H – Director Pediatric Palliative Care:
Talking with kids takes a lot of courage.

When they ask me the tough questions like "Am I going to die?" my first response is "Umm" and a deep breath, which gives me time to think and settle my heart down.

Then I say, *"That is really an important question. I wonder what made you ask that?"*

I let them then talk and I listen. It helps me to get on their tangent.

David S – Director Pediatric Palliative Care:
- Normalize the experience and layout range of options from other cases. Put conversation in the third person to depolarize the relationship and decrease tension with this family. So, you may say, some choose x, others y and still others z in such circumstances. This helps family look at the range of possibilities without it being too stressful or painful to them since it is not directed at them (no "you").
- Palliative care is the third leg of the stool represented by the patient/family and the primary medical service. Three legs provide more stability in the relationships and reduces the natural polarization that occurs when there are only two parties involved.

- To help families understand the reality of life closure I speak about my belief/observation that each of us comes into this world to learn lessons and to teach others through our relationships with them. I then ask if the parent feels as if the child has touched many others in his/her short lifetime. (They typically say, "Absolutely!") I follow that question up by asking what lessons the child might have come to learn and whether he/she has learned what she needed to in this lifetime?
- I say a prayer," May this child take only goodness as he passes from this life that will serve his soul, and leave behind pain and suffering that no longer serves the soul."

Eileen L – Pediatric Hospice Nurse:
- Although hospice work is sad, the joy I have experienced outweighs the sadness. We are privileged to get to know the patients and their world in a special way. It is an honor to be able to celebrate the child along with the parents. They do really help us learn to live in the present. It is a humbling experience to watch how much effort these parents put into their love and caring for the child.
- It is our job to support them, they are comforted by our entering into the hope they have, even as it changes over time.

- Guide them in their decisions. Listening is most important, they will tell us where they are and what they need from us. Helping them achieve some of the things they dreamed of doing with their child can help parents move to letting go.
- I have learned gratitude from parents, for the time they have had with their child.
- I no longer have fear of death. It is a peaceful natural transition to another phase of being. It has been a spiritual journey. Each life is complete in its own time. There is not much we can do to alter that but hopefully ease the transition.

Susan W – Hospice Bereavement Counselor:

Things to do for a patient that would help ease bereavement afterwards:

- Feeling that they did everything possible for the loved one to get better, to have the support they needed, and to feel as comfortable as possible.
- It is important for the family to feel that they had some quality time with their loved one prior to the death.
- In the case of children, sometimes it is helpful for the parents to meet other parents with a child with similar illness. These connections can be deep and are helpful later in bringing meaning to their lives by getting involved with community activities like fundraising for the specific illness.

- Memorialization is important and efforts to create new memories at the end of a loved one's life can soften bereavement as well.

Avis H – Hospice Chaplain:
Before I enter someone's home or before I begin a conversation that I know might be difficult or intense, I walk myself through a short exercise of slowing my breath and calling upon a spirit of goodness to rest with me. In calling this spirit I remember that I am not alone. I believe that if I listen well and am thoughtful in my own words and actions, this spirit will fill in wherever I am lacking – in sight, in courage, in strength or in wisdom. I have used this exercise (or one might call "prayer") professionally as a way of preparing myself and at times, I have suggested its use for our patients and our patients' family members. Sometimes it's only our fear of not knowing what to say that makes us not know what to say. Sometimes it is our preoccupation with ourselves that makes us stumble in these difficult conversations. This exercise makes me calm and peaceful, which in turn allows me to put my full attention to the task at hand.

James D – Nurse Team Manager, Pediatric Hospice:
- Over-communicate with your team. Do not assume everyone will get the message or the important issue of the day.
- Actions speak louder than words. It's the small things you do for a patient and family that

convinces them that you really care.
- Find the medical cocktail that makes even the most anxious client feel that "everything will be okay." This cocktail may include a combo of integrative and medical therapies such as favorite music in the background, cat on the bed, and some around the clock Haldol ...in one glass.
- Pain is the great energy robber and distractor. Manage the pain and the patient often becomes him or herself again.

Rene M – Hospice and Palliative Care Social Worker:

This is what I have learned really makes a difference in my encounters with others. To provide them with comfort and shroud them in warmth and peace, during a hard and painful time, I believe the most important things for me to keep in mind are:

- Every single family is bringing so much more to the room than we can see or know. They have rich histories, tapestries of events, woven into their souls. These unknown parts become instinctual nods to decisions that they ultimately make. It is only in truly listening and understanding the importance, do we walk with them, in making hard choices.
- When we stand in a place of judgment, we fail to see the reality for some of our most disenfranchised patients and families. That all of the things that this human being brings to their family is part of their reality. Sometimes this is the only caregiver of the young ones, the one whose

income means the added funds to buy groceries, have heat or electricity and not have to make the choice of which to have, the one that holds the adult children when they suffer or is the voice of peace and wisdom in a place of chaos.
- That to take the extra moment to create a place of comfort, warmth, and quiet and to offer and share a cup of tea or coffee, can make all the difference. To connect as human beings that are as alike as they are different. To show them in that moment of difficult discussions, that they are part of this fellowship of life.

Shahid A – Hospice and Palliative Care:
I thought I would add some of mine here as well:
- Making sure all the facts are clear to the key players.
- Clarity of diagnosis AND prognosis AND progress of the patient is paramount.
- Building relationships is key.
- Learn to listen and empathize.
- The power of therapeutic silence.
- Caring presence you show goes a long way.
- There is a lot more to medicine than just giving medicine.

Give 'I wish" messages:

I wish I had better news for you.

I wish he had responded to treatments well so we could pursue aggressive management.

I wish he did not have so many organs failing. I wish we had a magical cure, but we do not.

31 | PHYSICIAN-ASSISTED SUICIDE/ PHYSICIAN-ASSISTED DYING/ AID IN DYING/DEATH WITH DIGNITY

It would be impossible to talk about end of life issues in this book without mentioning physician aid in dying, previously referred to as physician-assisted suicide; and euthanasia. I have personally been asked multiple times by patients or families to expedite the end.

In a personal small unpublished study through a questionnaire that I conducted of physicians in Maryland who were not hospice or palliative care physicians, about 26% had received a request for hastening death, 8% had complied with the request, 6% had acted in hastening death without being asked.

This tells me that physician-aided dying is going on surreptitiously, and some physicians must feel strongly enough that it is the right thing to do that they are willing to put their licenses on the line.

What is of additional concern is that 20% of the physicians indicated that they had denied adequate pain relief to patients for fear of death as a side effect from pain meds. This continues to be a source of concern from both the patient's and the physician's perspective, even though it is ethically permissible as "double effect" where the intention of pain control is prime. Fear of litigation and doing harm, as well as the uncertainty of ethical and legal guidelines, continue to perpetuate this unfortunate suffering of many.

Case Study

The veterinarian daughter whose mother was in a lot of pain from terminal cancer said, "We treat animals better than you are treating my mother. Why can't you just give her something and put her out of her misery?" Her concerns of better pain management were addressed, and the ethical and legal ramifications shared.

In hospice care it is probably one of the not so uncommon ethical issues thought about and brought forth to the practitioners at one time or another. It is good to have thought about it, discussed it and have a rational, reasonable personal response to how you would handle this issue.

Your patients will need assurances that their suffering can be allayed without resorting to these measures. I believe this is possible in the vast majority of cases.

Just like most other ethical issues, there is no black or white answer. A lot will depend on the circumstances. One needs to look at both sides. Oregon experience shows that the majority of patients asking for aid in dying and hastening death were hospice patients to start with.

You as a physician are under no obligation to participate. But you are obliged to answer questions and help patients with their suffering when they raise this question. Some calm introspection of your beliefs and learning about facts from others' experiences is warranted here.

In my talks to general public on Advance Care Planning, I am invariably asked every time about the process and legality of hastening death if the person may so wish in the future, especially if they get afflicted with dementia. I believe the fear of a poor existence with dementia is a source of great concern in most minds.

Euthanasia is illegal in the U.S., and I don't see it being legalized here for a long time to come, perhaps never. It has been allowed in some Scandinavian countries from time to time.

Physician-assisted suicide, on the other hand, is already legal in multiple states in the U.S. (Oregon, Washington, Montana, New Hampshire, Vermont, and California), and many other states are working towards it. There is a lot of interest in physician aid in dying by patients, and by others worried about the possibility of dementia and neurodegenerative diseases in the future. It is not necessarily the best solution, but the fear and interest are definitely there. Patients are looking for choice and the peace of mind that they have some control over alleviating their suffering voluntarily if necessary.

A detailed conversation with patients to understand their reasons, their fears, and hopes that have led them to this decision is paramount. Even when legal, it is not an act to embark upon lightly. Being legal does not necessarily make it ethical and vice versa.

Like any ethical issue, in the right patient for the right reasons in situations where there are poor alternative choices, one may very well support such an action. It is a matter of choice on a very personal level and its availability is a source of comfort and control for those patients who want access.

To mention Oregon again, experience shows that about one third of the patients who got prescriptions to end their lives never filled them.

It behooves clinicians to be well-versed with the laws in their place of practice. Of course, just because it is legal, there is no compulsion for a physician to participate in it if he/she feels morally against it. As an alternative, patients need to be reassured and managed such that they do not suffer and their fears are allayed.

"I may not be able to assist in your wish for hastening your death, but I can assure you that I will do whatever it takes so that the pain and any and all suffering is managed, and I will not abandon you. I will always be there."

A few things that would help in not needing assisted suicide or euthanasia would be:

- A) Good management of pain and all suffering, including emotional, psychosocial, and spiritual. Hospices are a huge help in achieving this.
- B) Continued support of patient and family.
- C) Advance care planning with all patients about end of life goals and wishes <u>early</u> in the game while they still have capacity to make decisions. (See Chapter 11, "Advance Care Planning for End of Life in the Inpatient Setting – "The Three Questions…")

AAHPM provides guidance on evaluating and responding to requests for physician assistance in dying.

Suffering near end of life has many sources, loss of sense of self, loss of control, fear of future, fear of burden to others and physical pain; though pain is not the main reason for asking for physician aid in dying.

Here is a systematic approach to evaluating physician aid in dying (PAD) requests as suggested by the AAHPM:
1. Determine the nature of the request.
2. Clarify the causes of intractable suffering.
3. Evaluate patient's decision-making capacity.
4. Explore emotional factors.
5. Explore situational factors.

Here are suggested initial responses to PAD requests:
1. Utilize open-ended questions to understand. concerns that led to the PAD request.
2. Respond empathetically.
3. Reevaluate and modify treatment of pain and other physical symptoms.
4. Identify and address depression, anxiety, and/or spiritual suffering.
5. Consult with experts in spiritual and psychological suffering when appropriate.
6. Consult with hospice and palliative care colleagues.
7. Commit to the patient the intention of working towards a mutually acceptable solution for the patient's suffering.

When unacceptable suffering persists, consider benefits and burdens of other **ethically acceptable alternatives:**

1. Discontinuation of potentially life-prolonging treatments when life is not meaningful to the patient in the present clinical state when there is no reasonable chance of recovery. Life-prolonging treatments can be either medicines or machines that are helping to prolong life.
   (See chapter 21, "Addressing DNR/DNAR.")
2. VSED – Voluntarily Stopping Eating and Drinking, if acceptable to patient and physician.
3. Palliative sedation, potentially to unconsciousness.

32 | BEWARE OF BURNOUT

We are only as good for others as we are for ourselves. Let us make sure we take care of ourselves and our home and work environment so that we are the best we can be for our dear patients and families. Hospice and palliative care clinicians (HPC) have a higher burnout (62%) relative to hospitalists (52.3%) and oncologists (44.7%) (Harrison, 2017 and Kamal, 2016). The main reason is the unresolved stresses, which may be interpersonal and work-related, including the issues of moral distress that are common in HPC work.

My only reason to bring this up here is to remind us all to look out for it, avoid it, take care of it. The better we are, the better work we will do. (3) Organizations have to have policies supportive of the clinicians to help alleviate some of the pressures. Mass General Hospital utilizes monthly closed-door debriefing sessions, especially after difficult cases focusing on personal responses, yearly bereavement services for staff, good grief and chocolate at noon, wellness series, and education on communication and having difficult conversations.
(Ref: www.theschwartzcenter.org/ourprograms/rounds…)

Some of the helpful techniques for personal care can include stress release by loud activity like singing and screaming, leaving work at work (turn off electronic devices), having a ritual for the day's end (such as leaving work shoes in the garage, putting on sweat pants, putting papers in desk and locking it, singing and playing harmonica in car), positive thinking, humor, volunteering, social and emotional support groups of friends, buddies (such as male golfers weekly dinner night out without spouses), neighbors, families. Self-care can also involve sports, exercise; hobbies like painting, music; meditation, and mindfulness.

Most of us probably already have a system in place. If not, I suggest these four steps:

1. Find yourself an end of work day ritual.
2. Work on an organizational strategy to avoid burnout.
3. Start care-plans for your Palliative Care Team.
4. Start on self-care plans.

(Alkema, 2008)

References:

1. Harrison, K et al. Addressing palliative care Clinician Burnout in Organizations: A Workforce Necessity, an Ethical Imperative.
2. *J Pain Symptom Management* 2017;53:1091-1096
3. Kamal AH et al. Prevalence and predictors of burnout among hospice and palliative care clinicians in the US. *J Pain Symptom Management 2016*;51:690-696
4. Alkema, K et al: A study of relationships between self-care, Compassion-fatigue, and burnout among hospice professionals. *J of Social work in End of life and Palliative Care.* 2008; 4(2):101-19)

33 | REFLECTIONS ON DEATH AND DYING

- *I am dying with the help of too many physicians.*
  - Alexander the Great

- *There is no cure for birth or death save to enjoy the interlude.*
  - George Santayana

- *The long habit of living indisposeth us for dying.*
  - Thomas Browne

- *Expect an early death---it will keep you busier.*
  - Martin H. Fisher

- *He who fears death, dies every time he thinks of it.*
  - Stanislaus Lesycynski

- *Life is the leading cause of death!*
  - Unknown

- *Life is a sexually transmitted disease that's always fatal.*
  - Unknown

- *Death may be the greatest of all human blessings.*
  - Socrates

- *If the rich could hire other people to die for them, the poor could make a wonderful living.*
  - Yiddish proverb

- *At times, the pain of living is enough to kill you.*
  - Shahid Aziz

- *I have never wanted to see anybody die, but there are a few obituary notices I have read with pleasure.*
  - Clarence Darrow

- *Everything comes to him who waits – among other things, death.*
  - Francis Herbert Bradley

- *The fear of death is to be more dreaded than death.*
  - Publius Syrus

- *Death is not the worst thing; rather, when one who craves death cannot even attain that wish.*
  - Sophocles

- *I am prepared to meet my Maker. Whether my Maker is prepared to meet me is another matter.*
  - Winston Churchill

- *Death is the wish of some, relief of many and the end of all.*
  - Lucius Annaeus Seneca

- *He will live ill who does not know how to die well.*
  - Lucius Annaeus Seneca

- *No Man enjoys the true taste of life, but he who is ready and willing to quit it.*
  - Lucius Annaeus Seneca

- *Death is not the worst that can happen to men.*
  - Plato

- *Life without the courage of death is slavery.*
  - Lucius Annaeus Seneca

- *This life of ours is a sleep...and when we die we wake up from the sleep.*
  - Ali ibn-Abu-Talib

- *The fear of death follows from the fear of life. A man who lives fully is prepared to die at any time.*
  - Mark Twain

I thank you for the important work you do, thank you for your interest in this humble book and now please go take care of yourself first…

THE TIME FOR COURAGEOUS CONVERSATIONS ON DEATH AND DYING IS NOW!

APPENDIX

MY END OF LIFE GOALS AND PLANS

NAME: _____

Date of Birth: _____

Address: _____
_____

1. You may prolong my life by artificial means (medicines or machines) as long as at a minimum I am able to do the following:

   a) Regarding my mental awareness I want to be able to do the following:
   _____
   _____
   _____

   b) Physically I want to be able to at least
   _____
   _____
   _____

2. All life-prolonging treatments are acceptable as long as I can be rehabilitated to the levels mentioned above in 1a & 1b; otherwise please stop all treatments, including tube feedings and IV fluids, except for those that will help me stay comfortable and not suffer.

3. If my heart or breathing stops, only resuscitate me if I can get to my minimum levels of life as mentioned above in 1a & 1b, otherwise please let me die in peace.

4. No matter what, I do not want the following treatments:
   a) Tube feedings in severe dementia.
   b) ---
   c) ---
5. I wish to die at home in comfort and dignity.
6. Additional wishes: ---

HEALTHCARE POA *(Power of Attorney for health-related decisions)*

If I cannot make my own decisions, I want the following individuals to make decisions for me keeping my wishes outlined above along with the doctor's input.

1. Name and contact info:

2: (in case #1 is not available)

My Signature..

Date...............................

Witness # 1 (name/signature/date)

Witness #2 (name/signature/date)

   Discuss your wishes with family, friends, POA, and doctor AND give copies to all.

   Bring a copy with you whenever visiting doctor or a healthcare facility.

   Carry a card indicating you have an advance directive & give info on who to call.

IN GRATITUDE

I would like to sincerely thank one and all who have helped me in becoming a better person and physician. And those who have been so helpful in this quest of mine to write about the work I love so dearly.

First and foremost has been the unending support of all my children and my family, especially the encouragement and guidance of my wife Jean; immensely helpful review by Anita Tarzian, and the tireless patience and expertise of my very talented editor Maureen Ryan Griffin.

Then there are so many of the patients, families, teachers, students, colleagues and mentors and experts that I learned so much from. A few are mentioned here by name: Diane Meier, Sarah Freibert, Chris Kearney, Fred Heldrich, Nancy Hutton, Grace Brooke Huffman, Steve Wilkes, Geoff Coleman, Barbara Andersen, Eileen Lee, Anna Moretti, Caren Glassman, Edmund Pellegrino, Diane Hoffman, Jack Schwartz, Lynn McPherson, Beth Morton, Brigit Krizek, Heather Silver, Debbie LaFond, David Steinhorn, Carlos Zigel, Sarah Bayne, Nancy Eddy, Rene Mayo, Avis Hoyet-O'Conner, Susan Wilensky, James Dent, the Hospice and Palliative Care Teams at Montgomery Hospice, Hospice of Chesapeake, Children's National medical Center, MedStar Harbor Hospital and Laurel Regional Hospital in Maryland. Multiple professional societies especially AAHPM, NHPCO, AAP and ASBH.

Peace

ABOUT THE AUTHOR

Dr. Aziz, who is board certified in pediatrics, medical management, and hospice and palliative medicine, has talked to patients and their caregivers about end of life decisions over a thousand times in the last twenty years.

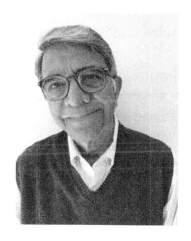

After graduating from King Edward Medical College in Lahore, Pakistan, he trained in pediatrics at the University of Maryland, Saint Agnes, and Mercy hospitals. He has been on the clinical faculty of the University of Maryland and Johns Hopkins, along with multiple local hospitals in the Baltimore metropolitan area.

He served as Assistant Chair of Pediatrics at Saint Agnes hospital, then Chair of Pediatrics and the Ethics Committee, as well as the VPMA at Medstar Harbor Hospital, all in Baltimore, Maryland.

Dr. Aziz was instrumental in helping start the pediatric hospice services at Hospice of Chesapeake in Maryland and the Palliative Care Program at Laurel Regional Hospital in Maryland.

He continues to chair multiple ethics committees, as well as serve on hospice/palliative care teams at local hospitals and at Montgomery Hospice in Rockville, Maryland, helping take care of children and adults. He is also actively involved in the education of the public and medical personnel.

Dr. Aziz has simplified the end of life decision process as a result of his active problem solving and crisis intervention for the terminally ill. Children and their parents, as well as adults, benefit from his thorough, efficient, succinct, and simple approach to making the end of life experience peaceful and meaningful. His mindful attention to personal needs, cultural and religious backgrounds, and family dynamics have produced an approach that is most beneficial to all concerned.

Understanding his model and following this thoughtful and thorough process will give professionals confidence, and their patients and loved ones peace of mind.

His book will help give the "gift" of peace to patients, their loved ones, and all serving on the end of life care team.

Made in the USA
Middletown, DE
21 April 2022

64383416R00126